MAC[illegible] DEGENERATION

A guide to help someone you love

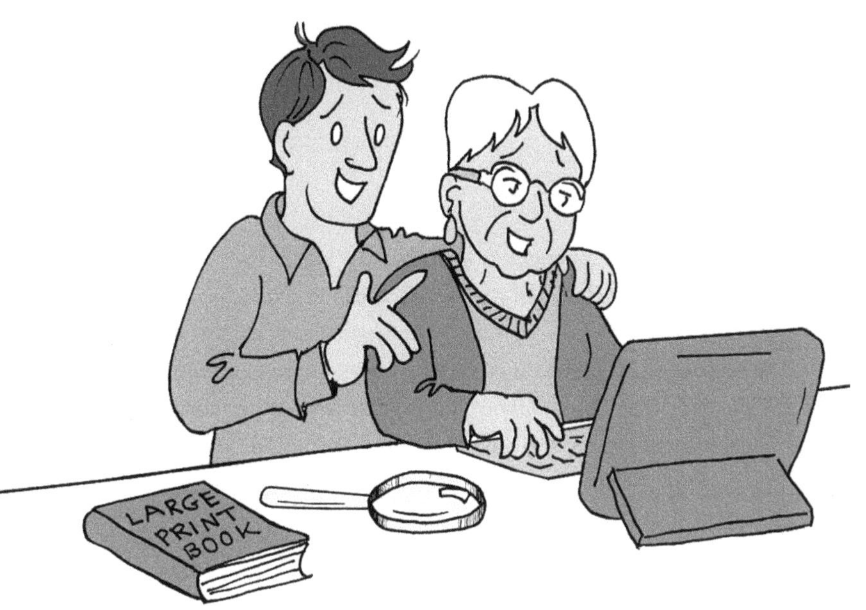

The book they need, but can no longer read

PAUL WALLIS

Printed in the United Kingdom

First Printing, 2018

ISBN 978-1-9995882-0-5 (Paperback)
ISBN 978-1-9995882-1-2 (eBook)

Paul Wallis
Riverview, Orchard Street
Dorchester, Dorset
DT1 1JY
United Kingdom

Foreword

Macular degeneration is the number one cause of blindness in the developed world. This book is designed for anyone with a family member, partner or friend who has lost vision to the disease. It will explain how you can help them to regain independence. I wrote this book for the people who surround the sufferer, who would like to help but do not really understand what is going on.

The first half of the book is the background information you need in order to gain that understanding, while the second half details more practical help for particular problems.

Over my career I have dealt with thousands of people with macular degeneration, and sought to solve their difficulties in coming to terms with visual loss. This is an area that is sadly neglected; much more energy is expended on diagnosis and treatment of the disease.

Becoming blind is one of the things we fear the most. I have attempted to explain why this fear is just that: a simple fear. Living with visual loss is a straightforward learning process when you understand the steps and previsions you need to take.

I hope this book will be the start of a successful journey for both you and your loved one. I have been on a journey myself in creating it: I am not a natural author and my journey to get this book to you has entailed much learning on my part. I am grateful to have met many helpful people along the way who have taught me new skills, ideas and techniques.

For trying to teach me writing skills, invaluable advice on this book's structure and for editing it, I owe Angharad Hill much gratitude. For checking technical points, my old colleague David Edgar, Emeritus professor, City University of London. Very special thanks go to my old student friend, Kevin Oxlade, who contributed his random and relevant thoughts, but particularly his personal story, and especially his wonderful illustrations. To Sam Pearce from SWATT Books for actually creating and publishing this book. To the late Janet Silver of Moorfields eye hospital, who taught me about LVA as a callow postgraduate. To my great aunt Phyllis, who inspired me by her work with deaf and blind girls in the East End of London through the Blitz of the Second world war.

The contributors I have to thank the most were all those people with MD whom I have met over the course of my career, who have taught me through their conversations, stories and experiences. I hope I may even have helped some of them as they will now help you. Finally, my thanks to my wife for putting up with my mental absences over the past few years as I tried to get my ramblings down on paper.

Contents

PART ONE

Faith is taking the first step even when you don't see the whole staircase

– Martin Luther King

Now all she does is sits or sleeps !
PHOTO ALBUM
BIN
BONESHAKER

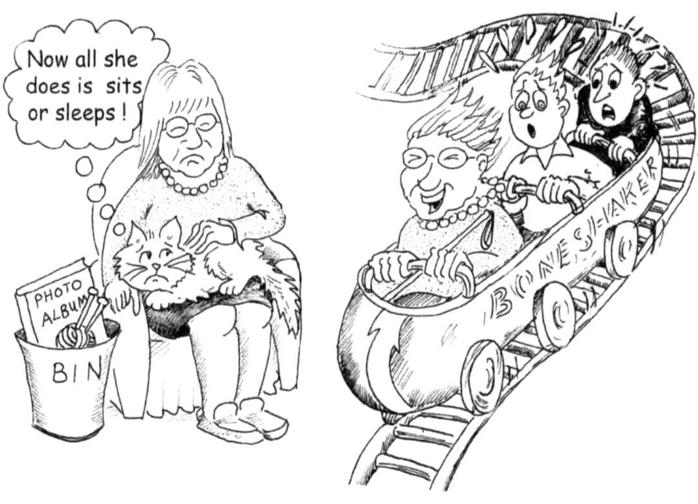

CHAPTER 1

Introduction: How This Book Works

Thirty years ago, I was working at Moorfields eye hospital in London as an optometrist. One afternoon a lady came to see me on her 90th birthday. She was confident the LVA (Low Visual Aid) Clinic was going to restore her vision, so that she would be able to resume her life as it used to be.

If you were selecting a grandmother by mail order, she was who you would pick; friendly, grey-haired, intelligent, with a sense of humour.

She wanted to read letters from her family, to keep her independence by going shopping and doing her own cooking.

The case seemed straightforward. I set to work and did what I had been taught. I got the information I needed, made an assessment and worked out how to help her. But in the process, I discovered her condition was just a bit too advanced and that my efforts were in vain.

She wouldn't be going home able to read her correspondence or to do her shopping with ease. There was an embarrassing moment where we both fell silent. We both realised I couldn't help. She stood to go, and thanked me graciously.

There was a sadness beneath the surface that neither of us could bear to acknowledge. I might have been the expert, but I felt incompetent. I hadn't helped. Her birthday was not a success. My faith in my job and abilities were dented by this incident.

They were further eroded over time. I saw people and supplied them with magnifiers; I would be politely thanked and they would go home. But a few weeks later I would notice that the magnifying glasses were quietly returned, as they were no use (though, 'they might be useful to someone else').

I wasn't addressing people's problems. The standard formula I'd been taught didn't seem to work for a significant number of the people I saw.

I left the London hospitals and went into independent practice in rural Dorset. I continued to see people on a scheme set up by the local NHS for the blind or partially sighted.

The work was different in the country. In London hospitals, you rarely saw the same patient twice, let alone more often. In London, there was little follow-up on an individual's progress. People just disappeared. In the country, you built up a bigger picture.

I began to see the long view. I often knew patients before they had visual problems. I saw them through crises and then afterwards, when they had weathered them. I gained a perspective on them as human beings and how they coped with the changes in their lives. They weren't just pairs of eyes.

Some didn't respond particularly well and some were challenging to deal with. The majority of people I saw for low vision work had macular degeneration. They were not part of the workload; they were the workload.

I almost gave up working with the blind and partially sighted. Disillusioned, I felt I was not helping. But then, as a result of spending cuts I came under moral pressure from the local hospital to see more cases.

As my workload increased, I changed my approach. I had the benefit of more experience, and nobody breathing down my neck. I was more relaxed. I began to listen and to watch people more closely.

I knew I was helping a bit, but there was more I could do. It has taken me 30 years to work out how to give that help, and to understand what is happening when an individual has sight loss.

This book is my atonement for failing that lady on her 90th birthday. I didn't understand what was going on. What I failed to do was give her hope for the future. I now know how to give that hope. That is what you, too, can give to the one you love by reading this book.

If you are reading this, it is because you have suddenly found yourself interested in a disease you know little about. A family member or friend has developed problems with their vision. This is traumatic for them and distressing for you. I am sorry for them, and for you.

The person you love who has macular degeneration is a very important person for you – a **VIP** in fact – but a **V**isually **I**mpaired **P**erson for the rest of the world. For the purposes of the book, I will refer to someone with macular degeneration as a VIP. He or she[1] is special and needs special treatment.

Your VIP will need your support and help in coming to terms with a frightening new world. You are to be congratulated for reading this. You can tell him about the disease and help implement some changes in his life.

Without your help, he is likely to curl up into a ball and retreat from life. With help, he can get back to being himself again.

As a friend of mine puts it, he can either mope or cope. Without help, most people will end up moping.

Giving help is a two-way street, however. You will be surprised how much you yourself can learn and change as a consequence. It should be win-win for both of you.

Most people assume eye-care professionals will provide the advice needed to cope with visual loss. An eye clinic will provide important information about macular degeneration. Indeed, a Google search will yield lots of information, but this information will take the form of facts about the disease.

It is more difficult to learn how to live with the consequences of visual loss. This book is not directly about the disease process of macular degeneration. It is about the **person** who has macular degeneration and how he is affected by the disease.

It should fill in the answers to the questions about how to cope with macular degeneration. After all, if you don't understand what is happening, it is difficult to know how to help. (I will explain details of the disease where necessary, though hopefully with as little jargon as possible.)

---

1 Please note that in the interest of total inclusion, this book will hereafter alternate between masculine and feminine pronouns chapter by chapter to ensure an easier read. In these instances we are always referring to whomever your VIP is regardless of gender.

The onset of macular disease can be sudden and traumatic, or it can tiptoe in over a long period. When it starts, friends and family are often unsure of what is happening. It may be dismissed as 'nothing important' or it may become a major issue, causing your VIP to fear for the future.

When the individual hits a crisis point, however, it will be obvious. He will no longer be able to do everyday tasks. This book has been written for just that crisis point, when the VIP's life seems to be collapsing about him. He can no longer drive. He cannot read a book, a newspaper or a gas bill. He cannot recognise you from a member of the public walking down the street.

Blindness is multi-faceted. There are, unfortunately, many different ways in which you can lose vision, macular degeneration being just one. Glaucoma, retinitis pigmentosa and corneal diseases all cause different forms of sight loss. This book is dedicated to macular degeneration, which has very specific characteristics.

Macular degeneration has been the leading cause of blindness in this country for the past one hundred years. But it was the unknown disease for most of the 20th century. The public just accepted that vision faded away as you got older. They didn't know why, or the name for the condition. The words 'macular degeneration' might be briefly mentioned in a hospital but the disease was rarely elaborated on.

Until the late 1990s, one visit to an eye clinic was all that was deemed necessary for most people. Once the diagnosis of macular degeneration was confirmed, the VIP was left to cope as best he could, with no further help. There was no treatment of any kind available. At best, it might be suggested he see the Low Visual Aid clinic.

Patients with macular degeneration were easy to deal with in hospitals. They were never hysterical. Often they were apathetic. They meekly hoped the professionals would relieve their problems.

When I trained, the procedures for macular degeneration were straightforward in the clinics. The routine was quick and efficient. It needed to be. There were large numbers of cases continuously arriving through the doors.

To be honest, they weren't the most exciting of cases. The patients were old and the attitude tended to be simple. *Suggest better lighting. Give them a magnifying glass.*

For the eye-care community, macular degeneration was not a sexy disease. There were lots of other forms of blindness where you could make more obvious progress and provide help. Younger people who had much greater life expectations and motivation.

There are fashions in diseases, and macular degeneration was not high fashion. That has begun to change over the past 15 years. It is now getting attention, for the first time, really.

It has always been the Cinderella of the eye-disease world, which is tragic considering it is the largest cause of blindness in the UK.

If you only have your VIP to deal with, it is difficult to understand what is happening to him and why. My hope is that by reading this you will be able to short-circuit what took me 30 years to understand.

This book should give you a wider appreciation of what happens when sight is lost. It will help you become a coach to give your VIP back his life. Too often the affected individual thinks his life is over. He believes he has reached the fag-end of life and simply gives up.

I truly believe this is not the case. Your VIP just needs some help to get him back on his feet again.

Julie's story

Julie came to see me with her mother for a consultation. Her mother was 77 and had been diagnosed with macular degeneration about six months before. She had been registered partially sighted and was living alone in a retirement warden-assisted flat. Julie lived about 80 miles away, and had a couple of teenagers about to leave for college. She was worried about her mother, who was only just coping on her own, having been widowed a few years ago.

They had a fractious mother-daughter relationship. Julie would often end up shouting at her mother, as she wouldn't do what she was told. The mother was retreating into herself and was getting very depressed and feeling cut off. Julie would come down once a month to take her mother to the hospital to get injections in her eye and would then rush off to do a month's shopping. Neither of them was enjoying themselves.

They were both ignoring the elephant in the room. Julie's mum was going blind and neither of them knew what to do to cope with it. They were trying to carry on as if nothing was happening. They were frightened of the future and didn't know how to deal with the now. Neither would admit her fear to the other, and lots of problems were being repressed but were popping out at odd moments, causing the arguments.

I couldn't solve all their problems, but I could explain them and impart some information. I lifted some weights from both women's shoulders during our consultation and they were happier when they realised there can be a return ticket with macular degeneration rather than just a one-way trip.

With information about how macular disease impinges on life, you will be able to make things very much easier for the person you love. In the process, your life will also change for the better.

To get the best out of this book, I would recommend you read all of Part One. This explains the what, how, why, where and when of the effects of macular degeneration – on the person, not just his eyes.

When you understand the background to the disease you will know how to help your VIP.

The second part is more specifically about how to help someone with visual loss, a way to think about coaching him back to an independent life.

The third part is about the various different areas of your VIP's life, with their specific problems. Not all of these areas will be a problem for everyone, but each individual is likely to need something from each chapter.

You may want to go straight to a particular chapter, but I would stress that to really help someone, reading through all of Part One will be the most beneficial, for both of you.

This book is for you, but there is a companion piece which is an audio book version for the VIP, it is designed specifically for them and is consequently slightly different, they don't need to know how bad their vision is they are living with it.

When you have finished reading this you may want to get them to listen to the audio version.

KEY POINTS

- There is hope after macular disease. The individual can become independent again.
- Macular disease is not the end of someone's life.
- Read all of Part One to understand how your VIP has been affected by visual loss.
- Dip in to Part Three as you feel necessary for specifics.
- Part Two is there to suggest strategies and information.

I can't wave a magic wand and solve all your VIP's problems, but I can give you practical advice and tips on dealing with common difficulties.

You are not the first to have trodden this path and you won't be the last. Learn from those who have been here before you. You don't need to re-invent the wheel.

You are <u>very important</u> and can make a real difference.
Thank you for reading this book. Good luck.

Science without religion is lame,
religion without science is blind

– Albert Einstein

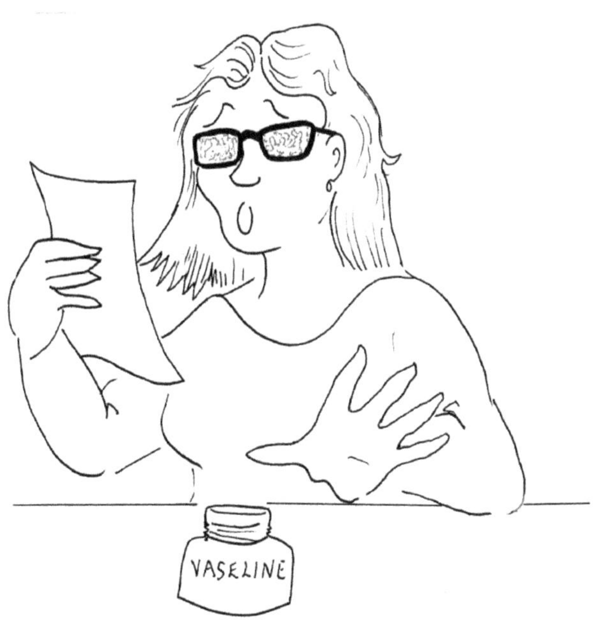

CHAPTER 2

What Is Macular Degeneration?

To make life easier for both of us, I will use the abbreviation MD throughout this book to stand for macular degeneration in all its forms. You may come across macular degeneration described in other literature as ARMD, Age Related Macular Degeneration, or sometimes AMD. They are all the same.

The difficulty of MD, if you don't have it, is understanding what is going on. As a concerned bystander, you hear the words 'Your father/mother/friend is going blind, or has been registered partially sighted.' You are confused; he or she is pottering about, isn't falling over the furniture, is complaining about a bit of difficulty reading. What is actually happening?

How to experience loss of vision from MD

Rather than give you a long lecture about visual loss (that comes later), I would recommend that you experience it in its raw intensity.

A simple exercise to create the world of a person with MD will teach you a lot very quickly. You are likely to spend several hours reading this book. Fifteen minutes doing the following exercise will teach you far more. 'A picture paints a thousand words', as the saying goes.

Please do this exercise rather than just reading about it. This is the best way of learning about macular degeneration. It is the most important part of this book!

- You need a pair of glasses. It doesn't matter if they are yours or someone else's. Sunglasses are fine as long as they have a pair of lenses in them
- You also need a pot of Vaseline, butter or margarine
- Smear the grease lightly all over both lenses so they are completely covered
- There should be no holes in the Vaseline that you can peek through. You only need a light smear, but all over the lenses, please.

You are now ready to experience the world of a person with MD. Wear the glasses for as long as possible. Try doing some of your daily routine. Please be aware of safety. Don't try anything that is obviously dangerous. Driving to the supermarket is definitely not recommended.

Try doing some of these:

- Make a cup of tea
- Watch television

- Read a paper
- Prepare food and cook it
- Use a computer or mobile phone
- Use the bathroom

Go up and down stairs. Are they free of clutter? Do you have to check that without the glasses? How would you know the stairs are clear if you couldn't remove the glasses? Check your emails. Can you recognise people? Would you recognise someone in the street?

Please take your safety seriously with this exercise

This exercise will let you experience being deprived of your sight and what a 'blind person' lives with on a daily basis. Try doing it for at least ten minutes.

____

____

If you have just done the exercise, welcome back!

You will have discovered that you were not 'blind' in the sense that you were unable to see anything. You should have been able to move around fairly well, but you couldn't recognise objects around you. You were 'blind to detail'.

I am surprised by how emotional some people become after this exercise. I have had people in tears when they realise what their loved one has to live with. You may not have had such a big reaction. It may simply have been relief to get your vision back when you removed the glasses.

The big problem with MD is loss of detail. Why does this happen?

Now the lecture on vision and how MD changes it

We see with the eye, but the eye is just the first part of the visual system. The visual image on the retina at the back of the eye is received by the nerves within the eye, and converted into neural information.

The nerves transmit down the optic nerves pathway to the brain. The bulk of the information goes to the optic area of your brain at the back of the head, just above your neck. From this visual area the input is broken up, transported and processed all over the brain.

Think of the brain as a city with many districts connected by roads and highways. Each district performs a particular function and is connected to other districts by more roads and highways.

Your vision is transported all over this city to many areas. Certain districts deal with colour, face recognition, movement, memory, speech or reading. The whole brain is involved in sorting the visual information and shunting it around to the relevant area for processing and then reprocessing.

As a student, it was repeatedly rammed into my head that the eye is part of the brain, rather than an independent organ. Vision takes up to 30% of the brain's processing power in a normally sighted person. Loss of vision is not just an assault on the eye but on the whole brain.

If you lose all vision you lose 30% of brain function. The retina is 30mm across, or one inch in old money. The macula is only 1.5mm across in the middle of the retina, but it is the most important area, as it handles 80% of the information from the eyes.

Although your VIP has only lost detail vision, that is 80% of all vision. I repeat it to stress how much it really is.

Therefore, the brain loses 24% of its information when MD strikes (80% of 30% being 24%).

This means having macular degeneration wipes out a quarter of your brain's input. This is a significant amount of information. Losing it is similar to the effect of a stroke.

Macular degeneration is regarded as visual loss. It is much more important than that. It is equivalent to serious brain damage.

The psychological side effects of MD are the aspect of the condition which is least appreciated and where you can help recovery most of all. We will look at that in much greater detail over the next few chapters. It is the heart of this book.

How does the eye change with MD?

We need to appreciate what is happening to the eye to cause this major loss of information to the brain. What are the mechanics of macular disease?

The inside of the eye is lined with 30mm of nerve fibre layer. The retina gives us our vision. It records the images you see all day long. It is like the film in an old-fashioned camera, before digital cameras came along. The majority of the retina doesn't record good-quality images. It only registers light and dark, and notices movement.

The retina consists of two types of light receptor: rods and cones. The majority of the retina is made of rods giving low-quality vision. In the middle of the retina is the macula which gives the high-quality (detailed vision). The macula is the size of this 'o'.

The central macula area consists only of cones. As you move away from the centre of the macula there is a mixed area of cones and rods only a couple of millimetres bigger. As you move from the centre to the periphery of the retina it quickly dwindles to just rods. At the periphery of the retina, (the corner of your vision) even the number of rods is diminishing.

The rods and cones have different functions. Rods give black and white vision and movement detection, while cones give colour vision and detail.

When cones are destroyed colour drains away from vision, giving a world of 50 shades of grey. It's like moving from full Technicolor to a black-and-white movie as the disease progresses. Some people with MD find the loss of colour quite marked, while others are not so concerned by it.

When the eye is functioning correctly the macula area handles the majority of the visual information, the 80% visual input to the brain. When you have your eyes tested at the optician, you are using your maculae. How far down the chart you read indicates how well the macula is working. The rods provide the other 20% of vision, your peripheral vision, the vision that stops you walking into doors or people and that helps you notice sabre-toothed tigers.

The macula is the high-definition area of the eye. You are using your macula area at the moment to read these words. If you look up and around the room, the macula gives you the detail of your surroundings.

We expect to be able to see all day long in varied lighting situations: looking at moving objects, reading text, driving a car, watching the TV or a mobile phone. Your eyes never stop working if they are open. The retina works hard all day, all your life. From opening your eyes each morning until you close them again at night.

This never-ending stream of pictures across the eye needs a lot of blood products to process it. The retina has one of the highest metabolic rates for tissue in the body. It is serviced by a layer immediately underneath it. Metabolising photopsins from the blood for the macula and retina requires a lot of energy. When the cones are working, the waste residues of the processing have to be carried away by the blood stream.

Unsurprisingly, the system can break down after 75 years of 24/7 use. It is amazing that it manages that well for so long for the majority of us. Not many 75-year-old cameras are in constant use nowadays.

The disease process

When macular degeneration attacks the retina, it destroys the cones. The damaged area gets bigger and the destruction becomes more complete. The word 'attack' is misleading. It suggests an inflammation that can be caught. You can't catch MD. It is more that the tissues of the eye wear out.

There are two types of MD: wet and dry degeneration. The majority of people – 90% – have dry MD. The remaining 10% have wet MD. Although that sounds like a black-and-white distinction there is a lot of shading between the two types. It is possible to have both wet and dry types simultaneously, with either occurring first.

Dry degeneration

When dry macular degeneration develops, the macular tissue literally disappears.

The problem is that, over a lifetime, waste products build up in the tissue just beneath the retina. Instead of the waste flowing away in the bloodstream, a small amount of debris hangs about and begins to clog up the tissues. Over a long period of time this debris causes the metabolism of the retina to break down. The cells of the supporting structure of the retina then begin to die. If this carries on more of the retina dies and vision reduces. The macula has the highest nutritional needs of the retina so it begins to break down first. The central high-quality vision disappears.

The macula is particularly vulnerable. To give high quality of vision from the cones, their blood supply is limited by coming only from underneath the retina. The rods have a blood supply from both underneath and on top of the tissue. The cones cannot have this top layer of blood supply, or it would block the light to the cones themselves, which means they do not have a back-up supply system of blood.

Once the blood supply is interrupted, the macula dies. The underlying support structure to the macula withers away. It is not possible to treat it, as there is no tissue left to repair.

The best analogy for this process is a pair of socks. When I was a child, my mother darned my socks. My wife doesn't bother. It isn't because my wife is lazy. Years ago, socks were made of wool. If you got a hole, you could darn across the hole into viable material. Now socks are made of nylon-type materials. When you get a hole, the material has perished and there is no useful material to darn into. The macula perishes in a similar way. This is why dry degeneration can't be treated or cured at present. The tissue has literally disappeared so it can't be repaired or treated.

Wet degeneration

Wet macular degeneration is a different process.

The layers of the retina are again degenerating, but the culprit this time is the retinal pigment layer. This is the layer immediately beneath the nerve fibre layer of the retina. There is a build-up of fluid between these layers. A small bubble of fluid lifts the macula away from its underlying blood supply. When this happens there is often a sudden distortion in the images of things. The retina is being bent out of shape. It may cause a lamppost to suddenly develop a kink in it, or a window frame to look warped.

The injections that are given for wet MD are to relieve the inflammation that is happening, causing the bubble to occur. As the bubble deflates, the vision returns – as long as the retina has not become detached from the underlying layers of the retina for too long.

This is a brief description of the disease process in macular degeneration.

With a diagnosis, medical treatment needs to be ongoing with wet MD. Regular consultations should be attended to ensure that the condition is under control.

Unfortunately, it is unlikely that vision lost to macular disease can be recovered.

How the vision is altered for an individual

MD changes each person's vision in a unique way. It depends what retinal tissue has been destroyed and how much.

This difference in vision can be illustrated by going back to the Vaseline glasses. I asked you to smear Vaseline all over the lenses for the exercise. Imagine if you did it in a different way. Instead of covering the whole lens, dab the Vaseline once in the centre. This would replicate the earliest change in macular disease. If you then kept dabbing, spreading out from the centre, that is how the disease develops. But every body would create a different dab pattern.

With a gradual spread of dabs across the lens there will be a loss of definition of vision. If there is a large loss centrally, a hole may develop in the vision. This would appear as a black patch centrally in the vision with peripheral vision around it. If the vision is lost in a random haphazard process, there may be several islands of vision left, giving variable vision across the retina.

The eventual effect is that the whole lens is smeared with Vaseline, so you get a diffuse image of the world but are unable to make out any detail.

Tom's story

When MD strikes and vision is lost, the immediate reaction is to try to get back to 'normal.' When you break a leg you are strapped up or put in plaster, and in a few weeks you are back walking and running again. Losing vision to MD is different. There is no return to normal as it was.

Tom had been an electrical engineer all his life; his son had followed him into engineering. When Tom came to see me, his son was despairing as he couldn't solve his dad's problems. Tom had always been an inventive man with a strong sense of curiosity. He always had some project on the go with lots of circuit boards lying around on his work bench. Now he was listless, with no interest in anything.

His son was trying to help him get back to normal as fast as possible. This in itself was not helping. If you have a stroke, it may take months of patient work to get back to a stable situation. MD is similar; you can't rush it.

With better insight, Tom and his son managed to get Tom's mojo back. What's more, they found it an enjoyable challenge. As engineers they relished the problems thrown up by MD. Looking for solutions gave them a chance to do stuff together again. Once they understood the problems, they could work their way around them.

KEY POINTS

I strongly suspect that you read the bit about smearing the spectacle lenses with Vaseline or butter, but didn't do it. That's fine... BUT DO DO IT. I promise you I won't be bossy again, but this really is important if you want to help your VIP. The reason why this exercise is critical will become apparent in the next couple of chapters.

- MD causes detail blindness not total vision loss
- The effect of MD is similar to the effects of a severe stroke with loss of brain function
- Learning to live with visual loss is a slow process
- DO THE EXERCISE WITH THE SMEARED GLASSES. If you don't do it now you will probably dismiss the idea as superfluous

The mental effects of MD are the areas which are least appreciated, and where you can speed rehabilitation most of all. This is what we will cover in the next chapter.

It is the absence of facts that frightens people: the gap you open, into which they pour their fears, fantasies, desires

– Hilary Mantel

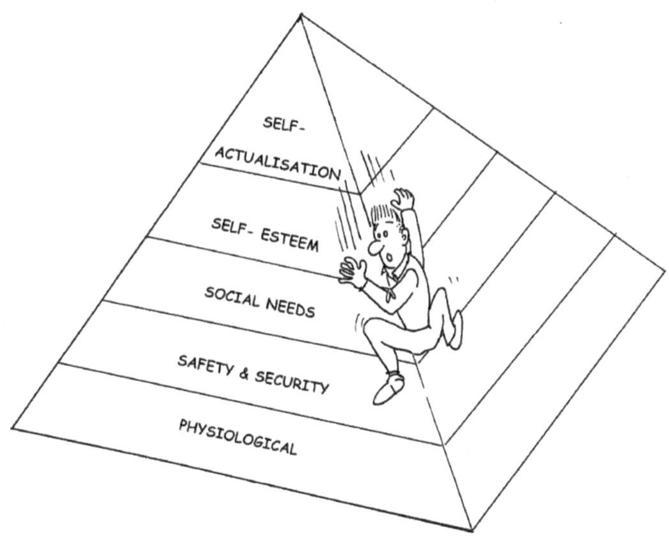

CHAPTER 3

Your VIP's Reaction To Losing Vision

Many people I meet are disappointed with their GPs or the hospital. They were expecting the medical establishment to 'sort them out' – to explain what has happened to them, what is likely to happen to them, how to cope with their visual loss and what to do next.

This is one of the big mistakes people make about the medical world. Medical professionals are interested in the disease. The aftermath of the disease is not their business.

The messy emotional aspects of visual loss are deliberately minimised by the hospital system. They may signpost people in certain directions if you are lucky.

They don't want people in distress causing havoc in a busy clinic. They step back and remain professionally detached. Language and discussions are carefully conducted in a low-key, objective way. It is often only on getting home that the patient realises she is going blind, having been told in a polite roundabout way that her vision is failing. The consequences have not been dwelt on.

This also applies to most of the books about MD by eye-care professionals. They are about disease process.

The diagnosis of MD and then the registration of partial-sighted or blind are significant moments in a person's life. The emotional impact is immediate. Short of being told you have terminal cancer there is probably no other diagnosis that will provoke such a reaction.

Blindness is often the number one fear that people have when they think of disability. That is why this book is focused on the consequences of MD.

If you lose a leg you can't walk, if you lose an arm you can't write – but it doesn't change who you are as an individual. You have to relearn walking or writing, but these are mechanical skills. These losses have profound impacts on lifestyle, but they don't impact your brain so directly.

Macular degeneration is thought of as a disease of the eye, but it is greater than that. It completely alters your life, and this is what people recognise and fear.

Lets follow someone after a diagnosis of MD

Mary is a practical person with down-to-earth common sense, rarely fazed by problems. She has been aware she was losing vision for some time before the diagnosis but she didn't realise it would be a permanent loss.

When given the news, she experiences two strong emotional reactions. The first is fear.

The word 'blind' is casually used by both the public and the eye-care community, but it has very different meanings for each group. The public understands blindness. It is simple. If you close your eyes you can't see anything. There is no light, no dark, no shapes, no movement – nothing, in fact, but total blackness.

The eye-care community has a very different understanding of blindness. It is technical, but they will register a person as blind when she can quite happily walk around as you did wearing glasses smeared with grease. The individual can't pick out detail, but she can get around on her own relatively easily.

Unfortunately, when someone is told she has MD, and is registered blind or partially sighted, this is often not explained – so Mary is expecting to lose all her vision, which is a very scary prospect. She has little idea how much vision she may end up with.

Visual loss from MD is virtually never complete loss of sight. In the trade we say that the person will always have 'navigational vision', which means she will always be able to get around on her own OK.

She can walk down the street without falling over benches or bumping into lampposts. But she could walk past her own son or daughter and never recognise them. She can't read prices, road signs, menus, or ingredients on packets.

If Mary has this properly explained – that she is not going to have complete loss of all vision – it immediately removes the frightening prospect of total blindness. She may still feel daunted, of course, and a lurking fear may remain for a long time, particularly where the loss is slow, and the worry is that the gradual loss will be unending.

The fear of total blindness is not justified. Your VIP is detail-blind. She will retain navigational vision.

Mary's second emotional reaction is grief. This is a very real, natural response to loss of vision and I would recommend that your VIP be allowed to grieve actively.

Loss of vision changes your life fundamentally. Activities, jobs, chores you took for granted, looked forward to or which were your raison d'être may no longer be possible.

Your VIP has suddenly lost the life she was used to and comfortable with. It is a devastating change. It is a death of her lifestyle, which is why it needs a period of grieving.

If Mary is lucky, a practitioner may mention to her the Kuebler Ross[2] model of grief. It is the only psychological tool I have ever heard applied to vision loss. The optical world doesn't traditionally concern itself with psychological problems.

Kuebler Ross's theory of loss was developed to explain what happens after someone you love dies, and how you cope and come to terms with it. It was taken up by the eye-care community as there are similarities.

Kuebler Ross's model states that the individual goes through five stages in the healing process.

These stages are:

1. **Denial.** This will go away. It won't be a problem. There must be a cure.
2. **Anger.** When the individual recognises that denial cannot continue, she becomes frustrated, especially with people around her. "Why me? It's not fair!" "How can this happen to me?" "Who is to blame?"
3. **Bargaining.** The third stage sees her trying to avoid the problem. This entails a search for a cure.

2 Elisabeth Kübler-Ross (July 8, 1926 – August 24, 2004) was a Swiss-American psychiatrist, a pioneer in near-death studies and the author of the groundbreaking book *On Death and Dying* (1969)

4. **Depression.** "I'm so sad, why bother with anything?" "I can't cope; what's the point?" In this state, the individual may become silent. She may refuse visitors and spend much of the time mournful and sullen.
5. **Acceptance.** "It's going to be OK." "I can't fight it; I may as well get on with life."
   In this last stage, she has come to terms with the change in her life.

These five stages are gone through to some degree by most people who have visual loss. For several years I used to ponder which stage a particular individual was at when I met her. I could never pin down exactly where she was on this spectrum of emotions.

Nobody ever seemed to fit anywhere precisely. They would be exhibiting bits of each level or none at all, or doing the stages but in the wrong order. They do go through the stages, but they may flip-flop through them. They can display different bits of different levels simultaneously.

This grieving process takes a while. Some people get through it relatively quickly. Others take years to come to terms with it. As a general rule, I expect most people to get through this period in about six months. It is not a steady progress through the grief, however. There are highs and lows and flashbacks to what life used to be like. Grief can suddenly flare up intensely if some incident triggers certain memories.

I struggled with helping people. I could understand the grief and the fear. These are what any human being would experience.

But there was obviously more going on than fear and grief. The change in someone like Mary after a few months was considerable. Undoubtedly, she was still in shock, and dealing with the grief of her loss. However, there was a deeper problem. She was a different, diminished person.

I would be sympathetic and empathetic whenever I met people suffering from MD. This was a primary need. But having given them some emotional support, when I then tried to move on to practical help, I often found I wasn't connecting with them. Something else was happening.

I began to realise that Kuebler Ross's theory has a place in the psychological pattern of what happens, but it isn't the whole story. There are other things going on.

I became quite disillusioned by seeing people with visual loss. I was doing the basics, but it wasn't enough. I couldn't put my finger on what was wrong. It took me a long time to work out what else was happening to the newly visually impaired.

The reaction I got from people confused me. I was offering help but the reaction to it was often negative or aggressive, or else I was met with apathy. It was difficult to get through to them.

They were rarely appreciative of my efforts. I began to reflect back their reactions to them, which wasn't good for them or for me. This was the point when I almost gave up doing LVA work, but was then dragged back into it by circumstances.

As I groped for an understanding of what was going on I came across another theory – Maslow's Hierarchy of Need[3]. Maslow was an American psychologist, writing in 1943. His theory was not developed with visual loss in mind. However, it translates fairly well to MD.

Maslow's theory of needs is often illustrated by a pyramid.

---

3 Abraham Maslow in his 1943 paper *"A Theory of Human Motivation"* in Psychological Review

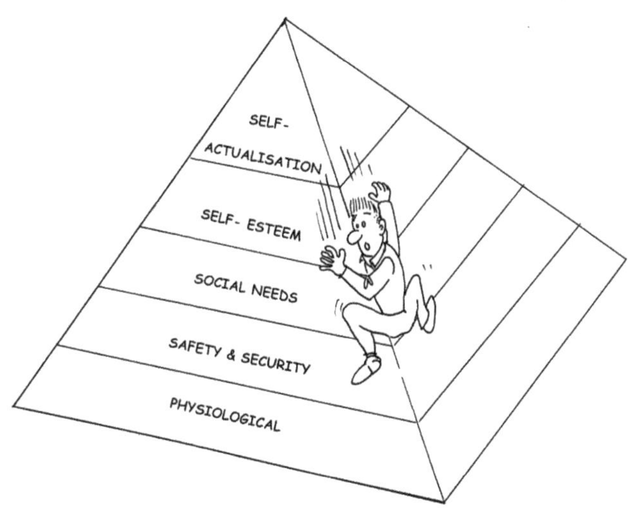

Maslow's Pyramid

Maslow assumed that people were trying to develop themselves throughout life. As they progressed they would gradually climb the pyramid, going from level to level.

Once one level of need was satisfied they would climb to the next. This would depend on them finding what they needed, within themselves or from the world.

They could climb or slip back from any level at any time depending on circumstances.

The foundation of the pyramid is the basic physiological level. We all need to function at this simplest level. Maslow explained this as breathing, having shelter, clothing, food and sleep. As children, these basics are provided by our parents.

Assuming we have the basics, we climb to the second level. Maslow regarded the second level as safety and security, which is all we need to know for our purposes.

The third level is associated with social needs. Being within group settings; loved within a family, as a member of a social/club group, a professional organisation, religious group, or by colleagues in a work setting.

The fourth level is the individual's need for self-esteem and self-respect. We want to feel valued within society. We want some degree of acceptance of our contribution to our social group within the world.

The final level is self-actualisation. This level of need refers to what a person's full potential is and the realisation of that potential. Maslow describes this level as the desire to do everything that one can, to become the most that one can be. He believed that only one in a hundred people would ever attain this level.

This model shows how one functions in the world. It is often a progression through life; the older you get the more levels you ascend.

Maslow and visual loss

Before vision loss happens, the individual will have been functioning at one of Maslow's five levels.

- She may have been a Nobel-prize-winning, fully self-actualised person, living at level five, the peak of the pyramid
- She might be your average pensioner,
  pottering around at level three
- At level one, she might be a chronically disabled person, functioning at the basic level of physiological needs

When MD strikes, the visual loss will knock the affected individual back to the bottom of the pyramid, to the physiological need of level one. Your VIP is now operating at the simplest level. She is struggling simply to feed and shelter herself. She is back to a level she probably last experienced as a young child, helpless. It will have been a long time since she last operated at

this level. Returning to it is a major shock, causing a loss of confidence and self-esteem.

- Her physiological needs suddenly become paramount. She can no longer see. Her individual pyramid has collapsed.
- She no longer feels safe and her security is at risk. She can't distinguish between friend or foe. The world is suddenly a frightening, threatening place. She feels she is a burden on her family. She fears being rejected by them. She may be frightened about having to ask for help.
- She is suddenly incompetent at tasks she has accomplished with ease throughout life. Her self-esteem and confidence may be destroyed.
- She faces having to re-climb her pyramid from the bottom.

Maslow's model illustrates what has happened because of MD. The rug has been pulled out from under the VIP's feet and she is back to surviving. To conquer MD, she has to start climbing back up Maslow's pyramid. Her whole world has collapsed around her on a physical and psychological level.

Mary will have suffered this collapse. She can probably almost feel the bruises from bumping down the steps of Maslow's pyramid. She can only manage the basics of life. The stuff she could do before is no longer possible. The simplest things are now a physical and mental challenge. She has lost control of her life.

This is what Mary, and all of us, are afraid of when we think of going blind. How do you live life from here on in?

In this state, the brain goes into a form of meltdown when trying to do normal tasks and activities. Self-esteem and confidence are shaken. The VIP's sense of self is radically altered. Her relationship with the world, other people, things she took for granted – all are suddenly changed.

She is upset and scared. She can't see how to manage. The future seems bleak and uninviting. This is the direct effect on the personality. The individual feels almost literally lost.

She is no longer a confident person who can get on with life independently. She needs help for what may be the first time since she was a young child. The freedom to be and do what she wants is slipping rapidly from her grasp.

The reaction is different for everyone, of course, but the underlying pressures are the same for all. It can be a toxic mix, and it takes a strong person to weather it. The affected person can easily become a 'shut in,' rarely leaving the house.

This is not a state anyone should remain in. But understanding what is happening makes it easier for you to help prevent the affected individual from spiralling down into depression, apathy and isolation.

It is almost like a descent into madness. The brain won't work properly. The affected person has been robbed of her status and self-belief. She is fearful for a future which is not looking great at this moment. She desperately needs some help to pick her up off the floor.

She is reduced to being a defenceless, incapable child, who is struggling to come to terms with the world. This is a profound shock to anybody, and cannot be shrugged off lightly or dealt with in a few minutes.

KEY POINTS

The consequences of loss of sight to MD are:

- The brain often behaves as if it has had a stroke
- The emotional effects are grief and fear, but these are relatively temporary reactions
- The individual is reduced to a basic functioning state, similar to being a toddler

These three effects happen almost simultaneously when there is a crisis point caused by significant sight loss.

The next chapter will explain how to counter these reactions to MD. I will explain a model for you to work from. I will help you to understand what is happening and thus learn how to help your VIP in the most effective way.

The best vision is insight

– Malcolm Forbes

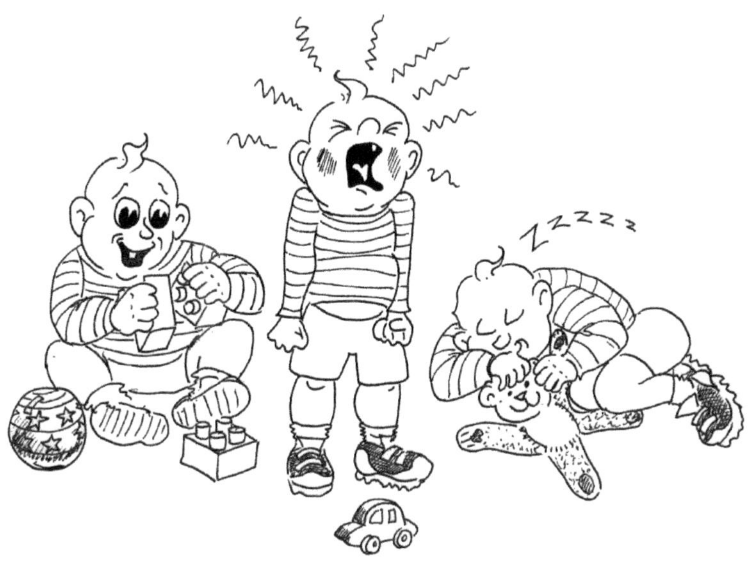

CHAPTER 4

How MD Returns You To Childhood: The Physiological Effects Of Vision Loss

How do the effects of grief, fear, and the loss of the ability to function normally change a person?

There will come a point when a line is crossed and your VIP finds he can't do something which is important.

He knew his vision wasn't right when the loss was only in one eye. However, it is not until the disease has caused visual loss in both eyes that real panic ensues.

When both eyes are affected, the situation changes completely. The Kuebler Ross model kicks in, while he simultaneously finds himself at the bottom of Maslow's pyramid.

What does it mean in real life? Think back to our Vaseline glasses exercise. What happened when you wore the glasses?

Immediately you were less sure of your surroundings and what was around you. Not too much problem at home, perhaps, but in a strange place you would be tentative; you would be unsure of what was around you. This is the first change precipitated by MD, a loss of confidence in one's ability to just be somewhere and a new uncertainty about what is happening.

Now let's imagine a trip to a supermarket.

When our vision is normal we walk into a supermarket and select a trolley or basket. We scan the store quickly to work out if it has been rearranged since our last visit, pick out the fruit and veg section, maybe note the display of mangoes on offer. Scanning the shoppers in the aisles to see if we recognise any friends or acquaintances, we set off up the first aisle.

Those actions take probably less than ten seconds. We know where we are, we feel safe and we know where we are going to go to get our purchases.

Ben's story

Ben lost his sight suddenly due to wet macular degeneration. He had burst blood vessels in both retinas which happened almost simultaneously. This is very rare in MD but does occasionally happen. He went from being a college lecturer to being a blind man with little peripheral vision in the space of two days.

Ben came to see me some weeks later with his wife and daughter. He told me about his recent experience.

He'd gone shopping with his wife at Asda. This was the first time he had been out since the loss of his sight. Keeping contact with one's partner is difficult at the best of times in a supermarket, and before long Ben's wife had darted off to get something from another aisle.

Ben found himself alone in the health and deodorant aisle, or possibly the grocery aisle. He couldn't tell. Which way did she go? Should he follow? Was there a one-way system in operation, unconsciously understood by customers? Ben could make out the cabinets and shelves but they were just a blur of colours and shapes.

The light made it difficult to see any changes in floor levels or whether anything had been spilt. Fortunately, Ben had the trolley to lean on; it was a 'comfort blanket,' but his level of anxiety was rising.

Suddenly a voice said, 'Hello'. Ben had no idea who it was or whether it was addressing him. He ignored it. His wife came back a few seconds later. Ben said he barely spoke on the journey home. He was so upset by the experience that he hadn't left the house again until he saw me.

Welcome to the world of the MD sufferer. It's a tough place.

Let's review what happened during that short trip to the supermarket.

Ben was running on adrenaline throughout the whole period when his wife left him on his own. His threat levels were high. He didn't know where to go, what to do. He was scrutinising all the visual information to try and get clues. *What's going on? Is the building safe to walk in? Was he going in the right direction? What is all this stuff around him? Did he know any of these people rapidly moving around?*

His brain was on fire. The amount of information he had to deal with was phenomenal. At the end of a minute of heavy neural activity, he was nowhere near as well-informed as a person with vision.

He was making assumptions and guesses about what was going on, weighing up the risks. Ben might as well have been in a war zone; it was that stressful.

Don't believe me? Put on the Vaseline-smeared glasses and try it yourself. The sheer fear of embarrassment will put you off doing that particular exercise. That stress you're reluctant to undertake is a fraction of the fear the MD sufferer has when out alone in public.

I don't generally like seeing people at Ben's stage, within three months of sudden vision loss. They are normally still very distressed. They are desperately seeking a return to their former state of being able to see – a perfectly understandable desire. They have to come to terms with the loss of vision before it is possible to help them.

The help will work best when the VIP recognises he has a problem. Until he accepts the visual loss – and that the loss is permanent – it is difficult to make much progress. If he can't accept the change, he will be deaf to most suggestions I or anyone else can make, being convinced he will get his vision back.

When he has come to a grudging acceptance that his vision has altered, he will have got through his initial panic. The grief for his lost lifestyle will be raw, but the implications will have begun to sink in.

The fear of further visual loss is still real at this stage, as the VIP's vision may still be changing.

Maslow's base level effect: a return to toddlerhood

What are the consequences of being returned to Maslow's base level?

We know the individual is operating as if he has had a stroke. His brain is working overtime. he cannot perform tasks that were routine and uncomplicated previously.

I came to call the effects 'the toddler syndrome.' This notion gradually took shape; it wasn't a blinding epiphany but, after mulling over the different behaviours of people with the same apparent problems, I recognised the patterns repeating themselves in different ways.

In short, the VIP begins to display a child's characteristics in an adult form. I nicknamed this 'the toddler syndrome.'

There are three parts to the toddler syndrome: **Tantrums**, **Tiredness** and **Play**.

I have used this analogy with hundreds of people over the years and found it useful. People understand it and can see its relevance. They recognise themselves and the insights it brings, and it is easily remembered (although initially people may be offended at being compared to a toddler).

The toddler syndrome

1. Tantrums

Anyone who has ever had to look after a toddler will recognise this scenario: a mother dragging a toddler out of a supermarket. It is one of the milestones of being a parent. The child has a meltdown – it either wants what it can't have or it can't do what it wants to do. The child proceeds to go into a full-blown tantrum, kicking, screaming and crying.

This is how the visually impaired person often feels. Due to his age, he won't disgrace himself in quite the way a real toddler does – but he will feel like doing so. His frustration is often just beneath the surface and will come bubbling up at all sorts of times. When he can no longer contain himself, he will have a grumpy patch. He gets overwhelmingly frustrated with himself, and often with those around him. He can no longer do all the tasks he has taken for granted all his life.

A few MD patients I have seen have been remarkably calm and controlled. The majority, however, have become much more cantankerous and grumpy. These feelings may be self-contained, but more often than not the grumpiness leaks out in their behaviour towards their nearest and dearest.

You may find yourself having to cope with a difficult person, even though grumpiness has never before been part of his normal character.

2. Tiredness

When the mother leaves the shop, with her toddler having had its tantrum, she is likely to shove it fairly roughly into its pushchair and set off up the road at a brisk pace, embarrassed by her child's behaviour. A hundred yards up the road she will still be fuming – but the child will probably be fast asleep.

The second 'toddler effect' is **tiredness**. Because the brain is working so hard, the new VIP tends to be exhausted. He will drift off to sleep at the drop of a hat. His energy levels are much lower than before the change in his vision. This is rarely acknowledged as a side effect of MD. Rather, it is often dismissed as simply a facet of getting older. The VIP *will* be older, true – but the tiredness is a direct effect of his brain being fried from simply trying to get through the day. He is genuinely exhausted because of the loss of his vision.

Don't forget, for MD sufferers a quarter of the brain's input has been lost. This is a severe shortfall of information. It forces the rest of the brain to go into hyper-drive to try to make up for that loss of information. This is the immediate physiological response to loss of vision. The brain is now desperately trying to make out what is happening.

Where, previously, the eye provided a clear picture of the world, which was interpreted by the brain, now there is a fuzzy image which has to be scrutinised and searched for clues and assumptions as to who or what is in front of it. The VIP's brain is working two to three times harder than the average person's.

With each and every task, the brain has to work much harder than normal, all day long. This type of mental work is exhausting. It is similar to trying to talk a different language all the time. If you have ever been abroad and tried to talk an unfamiliar language for a few days you will know how tiring it can be. Much like working on a computer all day, this type of non-stop brain work is exhausting.

At the same time, the brain is rewiring itself. It is still trying to function as before, but with poor-quality information. The normal pathways don't work anymore. These neural pathways are hardwired for vision and have been reinforced by many decades of use. As a result, the brain will now be searching for new, alternative routes.

Visual loss entails retraining your brain. There is no respite from it. The brain is working hard at interpreting the world. More energy is being used by the body. At a physiological level this is what happens with the descent to Maslow's base level one. **Exhaustion**.

This brain exhaustion has another interesting effect that, again, is often put down to age. Because so much processing power is now devoted just to seeing objects and working out what they are, there is little brain power left over for the individual to do much other thinking.

It is like having a computer with only a small amount of processing power. If you open up ten programmes and leave them running, there is not enough memory left for the processor to do any other work, so the computer runs slow.

It is the same for the VIP. When he has finally worked out what he thinks he has seen, he is often uninterested in doing anything about it, as he has run out of energy. Many VIPs begin to think they are developing Alzheimer's disease or that they are going gently mad because they can't get their brain to concentrate on much at all. This is a very serious worry to many of them, and they rarely connect it to their MD.

In fact, their brains are probably working harder and more efficiently than they have done for years. They are simply overwhelmed by the effort of trying to see, and by the fact that they are rewiring their neural networks.

Just being aware of the fact that he will be exhausted, that he is not losing his mental faculties, is likely to make your VIP feel a lot better about himself. So often VIPs think their symptoms of tiredness and mental slowness are caused by something else; they don't realise their symptoms are a direct result of their MD.

These two factors – frustration and exhaustion – limit the individual. They are the physiological response to not being able to see detail. They are the main problems that need to be overcome.

The good news is that both can be dealt with and eliminated by the process of coaching – which is where you come in.

These two symptoms of frustration and exhaustion can change a person quite profoundly. Your VIP may be tempted to shut down and not bother with anything. He begins thinking, 'my life is over'. The longer that state goes on, the harder it is to get him back to being himself.

There is a final component to the 'toddler syndrome' and that is what we will look at in the next chapter. It is the piece of the puzzle that completes the picture and shows the way forward.

KEY POINTS

Characteristics of someone with sight loss

- The toddler syndrome Part 1 - frustration
- The toddler syndrome Part 2 - exhaustion
- Your VIP may think he is getting Alzheimer's, or that he is 'losing it' due to lack of mental processing power
- This can lead to a loss of self-confidence and self-esteem

Life is what happens while you are busy making other plans

– John Lennon

Why don't we try....?
What if we.......?
How about....?
I wonder if....?
That is a good plan & ....
I am sure I am still able to....
eureka let's do it!
PAUL WALLIS
CVI

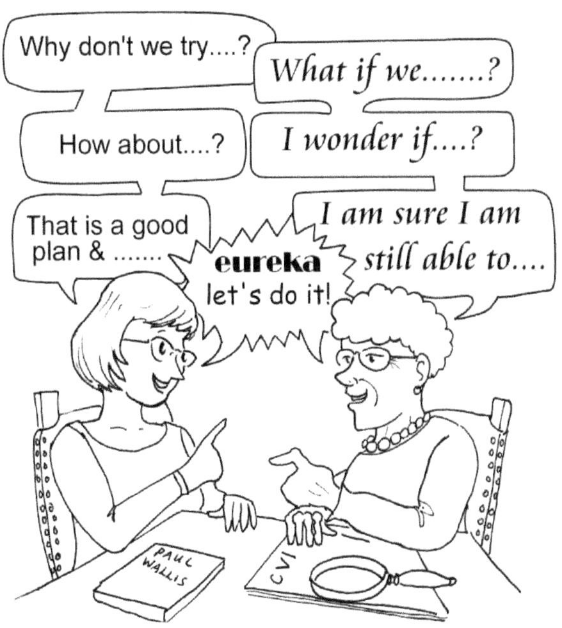

CHAPTER 5

The Final Piece Of The Puzzle (Toddler Syndrome Part 2)

If we accept that the VIP is dragged down to the level of a toddler, this is the clue as to how to get her back to being who she used to be – the final component of the toddler syndrome.

When the mother returns from her disastrous shopping trip she will let the toddler loose from the pushchair and it will spend the rest of the day playing.

Real toddlers spend the majority of their time playing, or that is how adults think of it. The child plays with objects, sticks them in her mouth, stands up, falls over, does all the things a toddler is meant to do.

When you think about it for a moment the toddler isn't really playing, however; she is *learning*. She is working out how the world works through play. It is interesting and fun. For her, the world is all new.

She spends hours doing not very much to an adult's eye, but in fact she is investigating, by observation and repetition, how to navigate her way through life.

When you have lost vision, you, like a toddler, must go through this learning period again. The normal assumption is that you just carry on with your life, but as we have seen, this causes frustration and exhaustion.

The MD sufferer needs to relearn how to do things from scratch. Play is the key to unlocking the exhaustion and frustration of vision loss.

There is one major difference in behaviour between a toddler and a VIP: their intentions. A toddler performs actions out of a sense of curiosity. She is not trying to get a result. She is interested purely in the process of doing something. As a result of play she may discover she can stand up or walk, but that is almost a side effect of her actions.

An older person is almost the exact opposite. She wants a result. She is not interested in the process. If she can't read the weather forecast in the paper, she gets frustrated. She specifically wants a result – anything that gets in her way is annoying, particularly when she has been doing something successfully for decades.

This is the source of her irritation. The processes she has been using for years no longer work.

The VIP needs to relearn how to do many tasks that have become ingrained by a lifetime of repetition. This repetition has also caused her to see her habitual action as the 'right way' to do something.

Any routine is a strong network pathway of muscle and nerve memories. Hopping in your car, turning the key in the ignition and backing out of your driveway can all happen without you even thinking about it. This feeling of being in control is a result of the brain's circuitry having been strengthened through repetition.

The problem for the VIP is that her brains are overloaded from trying to cope with a new world of poor vision. Her fall-back position is to rely on old habits, but these are failing her as she has insufficient vision. A classic Catch-22 situation.

This is why the idea of play is useful. If you can reduce the VIP's problems to a series of games or puzzles that need to be solved it is easier for everyone, and the ideas of failure and success are minimised because you are playing. You can't fail when you are playing – you just have fun, and maybe a laugh or two along the way.

The toddler is happy to bumble around, fall over, sit down, chew the carpet – whatever happens to appear before her at that moment. She has no plans to be a nuclear physicist. She just wants to taste, feel, touch, look at whatever is around her.

However, by a series of movements, endeavours, accidents and encouragement she suddenly discovers she can walk around on two legs like her parents. 'RESULT!' She then get lots of praise and cuddles from the people around her. The more she does the more excited her parents become.

The VIP, on the other hand, feels everything is being taken away from her, bit by bit. She can't read, she can't drive, she loses confidence in public... What she gets is sympathy and reassurance, but life feels like a downward spiral, which is positively depressing. No wonder she begins to inhabit this sad, depressed world that seems to be closing in around her.

While she wants a bit of tea and sympathy, what she needs is a positive outlook and some positive help to get her back into the saddle of life. She doesn't want or need to be told that it is all over for her now (which is the impression often given by well-meaning people).

Alec's story

Alec had been a plumber all his life, working 'on the tools' for 20 years before switching to teaching plumbing at the local college. Until he was 70 he was still enjoying teaching his 'lads'. When MD began to cause him problems he found he had difficulty marking work out, reading a tape measure and inspecting detail on students' work. Reluctantly, he gave up work.

When I saw him, he was still pottering around, doing jobs in his shed at home, though he now needed some help with the detailed work.

I explained 'the toddler syndrome', which he took on board and, having thought for a bit, this is what he said to me: 'When the lads turn up to their plumbing class on the first day they have some of the kit and they're very willing but they aren't plumbers after their first day. I suppose it is like that with going blind. You have to learn it.'

He was right. When you are training to be a plumber you are expected and allowed to make mistakes. Likewise, you have to practise being blind. It's a skill, and as you practise you get better at it. You aren't 'qualified' to be blind on your first day.

Every time you learn something new, connections form between neurons in your brain. The more repetition there is the stronger the electrical signal, the stronger the connection. The VIP has to build the muscle and nerve memories of new habits.

The main problem with this is that the VIP doesn't have much mental firepower – hence we have to tread lightly in our efforts to help. Otherwise she will get even more frustrated, and instead of helping, you will be regarded as a nuisance who is forcing her to do things she can't cope with. She will fight you instead of seeing that you are trying to help her.

You can make progress with your VIP, but it will probably be a lot slower than you imagine. A stroke victim can take years to recover some functions. With steady progress, you will realise she has made huge strides, but in very little steps.

It is frustrating for both of you trying to get somebody to do something differently from the way she has always done it. It is easy to get grumpy and frustrated with each other. However, patience is the name of the game.

The final bit of theory

What is going on when VIPs cling to old habits

An illustration of why we cling to habits is given by the work of Daniel Kahneman. Kahneman wrote a book called *Thinking Fast and Slow*[4]. His theory is that humans have two ways of thinking: 'fast' and 'slow'. As humans we will pick the fast solution to a problem in preference to the slow, not only because it is quick but because it is less energy-consuming. This applies to thinking as well as to physical actions.

We build up a series of habits or default ways of doing things that work for us. These require virtually no thought. We tie ties or shoelaces with no effort. We use lawnmowers and food mixers. Some of us can even operate a mobile phone without the help of a five-year-old.

If we had to explain how to tie a tie we might struggle to explain which bit goes where at which moment, and yet we have set up pathways in our brains so that the actual process is simple and performed with no great expenditure of mental energy.

4 Daniel Kahneman (25 October 2011). *Thinking, Fast and Slow.* Macmillan. ISBN 978-1-4299-6935-2

As an example of fast and slow thinking, if I were to ask you the sum of 2 plus 2, your reply would be fairly instantaneous: 4. That is fast thinking.

If, however, I were to ask what 73 multiplied by 57 is, I would be highly surprised if you replied as quickly, though you could perhaps work out the answer after some mental gymnastics and maybe playing with your fingers. Try it. This is slow thinking.

Once you have arrived at the second answer you may notice how tiring it was doing that exercise. You have literally had to use your brain energy to solve it. It is why the person using a computer is tired at the end of the day.

Because slow thinking is so energy-consuming, we try to reduce our daily life to a series of habits, which are examples of fast thinking. That is the purpose of childhood: we are creating a series of templates for patterns of behaviours that we can use in situations to conserve our mental firepower for the difficult things in life.

The problem for the VIP is that all her fast solutions have suddenly become useless. She is reduced to slow thinking all the time, which requires a lot of time and energy.

By utilising play with your VIP you are trying to give her new 'fast' solutions. Her previous fast solutions have changed with her loss of sight, becoming slow solutions, but she is only half aware of this.

How can we use play for your VIP?

Essentially, this is a process of problem solving. We need to look at the problems confronting your VIP and solve them one by one. Start with a simple problem and then gradually work through them.

There are three components to this:

1. Recognise a problem area, something that is causing her frustration and problems
2. Having found a problem, we have to do some brainstorming to think of ways around it
3. We have to instigate 'play' to set up a new process for the problem

Recognising problems

A big problem may be actually getting your VIP to admit to 'problems'. Often, she doesn't recognise what problems she has; her habits are so ingrained she can't imagine doing things differently. So a little digging may be necessary to uncover their frustrations.

Let's have a cup of tea

As an example, let's think about making a cup of tea. Most of us, if we are British, want to settle down with a cup of tea or coffee and relax at some point during our day – a simple pleasure of life.

However, if making the cup of tea is fraught with danger or potential disaster, the eventual cup may not be quite so welcome. The MD sufferer can all too easily make a mess with water, milk, sugar or tea, and there is also a danger of electrocution, burning or scalding.

Your VIP may not have a problem with this particular process, but we will nevertheless work through tea-making as an exercise to illustrate how to play with an 80-year-old.

A play session should really be done with another person, which is where you come in. For the exercise, the first thing to do is make a cup of tea and sit down with your VIP.

The second part of the exercise is about brainstorming how to make a cuppa easily, safely and without making a mess.

Over your cups of tea, have a conversation with your VIP about how to make tea. Try to come up with lots of different ideas, no holds barred. Think of as many bizarre ideas for tea-making as you can come up with.

When you have come up with many different options and techniques, you can discard the more outlandish ones, but you should be left with various ways which are different from your VIP's normal process.

When you have finished off your own cups of tea, trot off to the kitchen together to make a series of cups of tea in the different ways you came up with. You will waste a few tea bags and some hot water at worst.

The most important part of this exercise is making sure that when your VIP goes to 'make' tea she has just had some – therefore she doesn't need or want tea at the point of play. When she goes to the kitchen, it will be purely to play at making tea. She can concentrate purely on the 'process' of tea making.

Safety is paramount: be careful with boiling water and electricity/gas, but as your VIP has to live in the real world, these issues need to be addressed.

Part three: playing in the kitchen

You might come up with the idea of filling a mug up with cold water from the tap and then putting it in the microwave oven. Set the microwave for a certain amount of time, depending on the microwave, and then, when it goes ping, you remove the cup with the hot water in it, pop in your tea bag or instant coffee and bingo, you have a cup of tea (adding milk either before or after the microwave).

Sugar lumps rather than loose sugar? There are all sorts of variants. My son has a device in his kitchen that you fill with cold water; you switch it on and it heats the water like a kettle, but when the water is hot you press a button and it dispenses a set amount of water into the cup beneath it.

...

You could use a device which you rest in the cup and which bleeps when the water touches it.

...

All these methods work. They have advantages and disadvantages, but none will have made a mess or endangered anyone. You can try lots of different ways of going about it. You know what your desired result is – you want a cup of tea – it is just a question of how you get there. You are going to waste a few teabags some water and electricity, but don't worry. Have some FUN. Keep it light-hearted. There are no rights or wrongs, just what works for your VIP.

The point is to override her original habits of thought and create new 'fast' patterns of behaviour. It is easier for your VIP if this is done with another person to break up those habits and to give her positive feedback when she's successful.

The attempts may not be immediately successful but you can cajole if necessary and suggest different ideas until a new pattern is created. This is meant to be play, so no pressure should be put on your VIP. If the alternative techniques don't work for her, never mind, try something else, or just accept that the way she does it may stay the same for the time being. Nevertheless, seeds will have been sown for her future behaviour.

You should only aim for one play session per day and this session should be only a few minutes long. Your VIP will get too exhausted otherwise. But if you can solve one problem a day you can make surprising progress over a few weeks. You will also find you've got your VIP into a positive feedback loop where she can appreciate that she is regaining control of her life.

If the play session produces a solution to a problem, the next session can be looked forward to. Changing habits takes time and is energy-consuming, but eventually old habits can be changed to new ones.

You can motivate your VIP and make it easy for her to have the play session in a safe way. While trying out new ideas, do them yourself with the Vaseline-smeared glasses to see if you are asking too much of her. As it is a game, it may be fun for the VIP to see you make a fool of yourself – this may help her feel less bad about her own struggles. Although this game has a serious purpose, it doesn't have to be miserable.

MD is like a troublesome family member who questions her behaviour every time she tries to do something new. The old behaviour patterns are thrown in the air. They won't work right. It is too difficult. Old reassuring ways are no longer reassuring, which is distressing in itself.

Via play, we can give the VIP new habits that work, to give her back her equilibrium. She wants to be able to do 'stuff' without a tussle or struggle. New techniques need to become automatic, with little need to engage the brain.

The 'toddler' model I have outlined shows the problems, frustrations and exhaustion that can slow the process of adaption, and which often change the personality traits of the VIP. It also offers the key component – *play* – which can help her get back to an independent, stable life.

KEY POINTS

- Play is the way to change habits, if the habits no longer work.
- Solving problems for your VIP is mainly a thinking exercise
- Identify problems
- Brainstorm solutions
- 'Play' and try the solutions out
- Create new habits; fast rather than slow thinking is needed
- VIPs can only cope with one play session a day, so take care not to overtax them

Next, before we can get on with the rehabilitation process, we need to consider the person as a whole, as opposed to just a pair of eyeballs. What is your VIP's personality like?

We can easily forgive a child who is afraid of the dark; the real tragedy of life is when we are afraid of the light

– Plato

Macular degeneration is the thief of time - everything takes a lot longer !
I really miss driving
I won't be able to do my job !
I'm a fighter !
Why me?
I'm determined to remain independent!

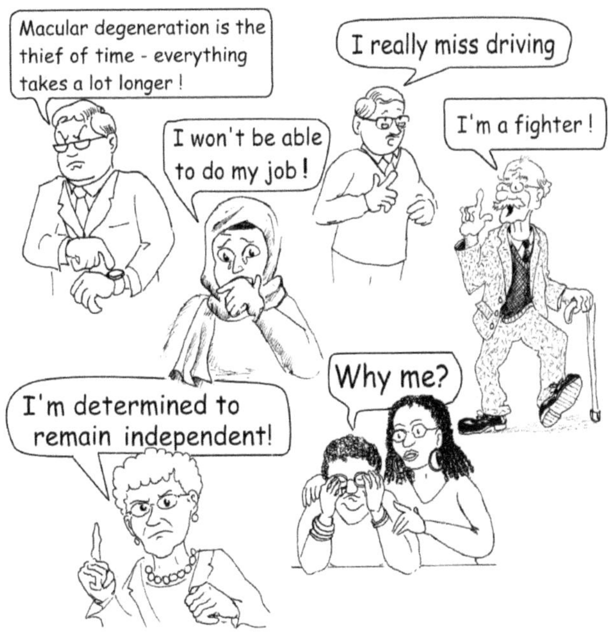

CHAPTER 6

The VIP As An Individual, Not Just A Pair Of Eyeballs

The 'toddler syndrome' model is applicable to all VIPs with MD. The frustrations, exhaustion and loss of mental processing are the same in all sufferers, as is the idea of play.

However, not all VIPs are alike. They are all completely different in their needs, desires and capabilities. What is going to work for one won't work for all.

Over many years I have seen MD affect various shapes and sizes of people, all of whom have widely varying personality types. It is difficult to give blanket advice on how to come to terms with MD, but there are common factors that will vary from person to person. You need to be aware of these when trying to help and be sensitive to whichever factors are dominant in your VIP's character.

The main characteristics that influence ability to cope are:

1. Age of individual at time of visual loss
2. Severity and speed of onset of the disease
3. Personality type
4. Physical/mental conditions apart from vision
5. How controlling is the personality?
6. Social factors
7. Motivation

Every individual will be a cocktail of these factors. They have to be teased apart to see how they interact, and what the implications will be on how quickly the individual can progress.

1. Age of the individual at time of significant sight loss

The younger the individual is when he loses significant sight, the quicker and more complete his likely rehabilitation. If he is under the age of 75, he will often cope very well in the long term. From 80 to 85 years old, sufferers may take longer to adapt to new situations. The over-85s are less resilient to problems, but can cope given enough time. However, at this age they often feel little enthusiasm for new challenges and may end up being quite passive in the face of what they see as an insurmountable problem.

Elsie's story

Elsie had always lived locally and her family also lived close by. She had three daughters with a selection of grandchildren and was about to become a great grandma when she was registered partially sighted.

She had been widowed a couple of years before, so when her vision started failing her eldest daughter swept her up and created a granny flat on the end of their farmhouse.

Elsie was 85. Her vision had been failing for a couple of years before it took a turn for the worse. Her daughter did all the cooking and Elsie was just another mouth at the dinner table. Her grandchildren took having her around as perfectly natural, and helped her out, when they could be detached from their electronic devices.

Elsie had a lot going on around her all the time, so she was happy to retreat to her annexe for some peace and quiet. The family kept her entertained and she was quite content listening to the radio and TV.

Her motivation was low. She was happy and content as she was, although she did want to be able to read the TV listings a bit more clearly.

2. Severity and speed of onset of the disease

The onset of the disease varies dramatically, from very gentle, over a period of years, to a sudden onset that can take place in as little as a few weeks. The 'slow' type often means the person adapts gradually to the change in his vision, hardly even aware the adaptation is happening. The TV picture isn't as sharp, and reading is a bit more difficult, so he changes behaviour patterns, while friends and family are often oblivious to any problem.

The 'slow onset' disease still reaches a crunch point eventually, however. Like a slow car crash, the VIP comes to realise he has a problem he can no longer deal with. The slow onset sufferer tends to be more phlegmatic; he has realised his vision is altering and is more prepared for the tipping point when it hits him. Being aware of the problem, he is not shocked by it, though his visual loss is of course still difficult.

When there is sudden and large loss onset, however, it can be much more frightening. 'Fast' visual loss comes with little warning. Panic often ensues and, for the VIP, there is likely to be frantic activity in an attempt to cure the condition. This is where Kuebler Ross's model is most accurate; the VIP must move through states of denial, anger, bargaining, depression and finally acceptance before he can come to terms with his condition.

With fast onset MD, it is often difficult to get through to the VIP initially, to help him understand what is happening and how to deal with it. If I see the sufferer at this point, I tend just to listen to him and let him vent his frustrations, as well as trying to persuade him not to waste too much money on the latest gadgets. The VIP at this stage is still convinced he can solve his problems and get back to the life he has lost and for which he is still grieving.

3. Personality type

I am often surprised by the reaction of people to visual loss. The majority of people go through the primary emotional responses of the Kuebler Ross model, denial and anger, followed by the secondary 'toddler syndrome' effects of frustration and exhaustion. These can combine to create a rather difficult old person.

Strangely, though, this sometimes doesn't happen. I have sometimes suggested to someone that he may have been feeling a bit crabby lately, only to be greeted with a genuinely questioning look and smile and the response, 'No,' from both the family and the person with MD.

'He never loses his rag or gets upset. He is perfectly happy.' It is true that there are some remarkably serene people in the world – people who are able to rise above the difficulties inflicted by MD – but they are in the minority.

There are thousands of personality types. Women's magazines are constantly bombarding their readers with surveys to help them identify their personality stereotype. We are all unique, but trying to analyse why some people adapt to visual loss and others don't is fascinating.

Introverts and extroverts react either positively or negatively. Introverts may retreat into themselves to solve their problems, or just retreat and wither away alone.

Extroverts may share their difficulties with everyone and seek help to solve problems, or they may use others to do things for them, avoiding confronting the issues directly.

The person who has been proactive in life and is a problem solver tends to cope best. If his job has meant he has had to solve practical problems – whether he was a car mechanic, a farmer or a scientist – he very often responds well to the problem-solving of visual loss.

If, however, the sufferer has been a passive individual who has not had to confront problem-solving, he may have trouble adapting. If he expects a job to be done for him, for instance, he may experience distress when someone doesn't come along and wave a magic wand to make his problems go away.

Alternatively, he may become passive, and actively enjoy the fact that he can't do anything for himself. After all, he is now receiving lots of attention because he has 'gone blind' and needs to be looked after. He may suddenly start seeing family members a lot more, and get sympathy and help. For certain personality types in this scenario, what's not to like?

The question of personality type boils down to, *can I fight this, and do I want to?* Your VIP may react either way. It is often a subconscious decision influenced by many factors.

When I see someone who needs help, I find I prefer it if he is a bit grumpy. It is more likely he will make progress if you can harness that dissatisfaction. If the sufferer is too serene he may not be bothered about the visual loss and, equally, may not be bothered enough to do anything about it.

Margaret's story

Margaret was the widow of a war veteran. Her vision had been poor for many years due to a combination of factors. Following the death of her husband, her diabetes spiralled out of control and, as a result of both diabetes and MD, her vision finally reduced quite catastrophically over a period of three months.

The mixture of personal grief, diabetes and loss of vision left her in a real quandary. Margaret was now living alone in a village with no public or personal transport. She was fighting on multiple fronts, some of which had arisen quickly.

The main thing in her favour was that she had always been a 'difficult' woman. She had been a union official all her working life. She relished a fight and wasn't going to take anything lying down. (In a bare-knuckle fight with Margaret Thatcher, the PM would have lost.)

MD was one of her hardest battles, but Margaret fought back and overcame the obstacles in her way. Within three months of her husband's death and the loss of her sight (which happened very close together), she had organised a series of lifts for herself into the town from the village where she lived, and had sorted herself out quite remarkably.

4. The physical and mental state of the person, apart from vision

John Donne's line 'No man is an island' is something of a cliché, but it's true. A person's vision is just one component of being human. We can't regard visual loss in isolation. We function on many levels. As we get older we accumulate a selection of physical problems that may be minor irritants or may be much more serious. Older people may even have terminal conditions in addition to MD; in such cases, a loss of vision may seem relatively unimportant.

We need to bear in mind the whole person and how much he is already dealing with. We have seen how fighting back from visual loss can demand great energy, both physical and mental. If the VIP is stressed by other things, his energy reserves are going to be much lower. If he has chronic pain – from arthritis, for instance – this is likely to be exhausting for him, and it may be restricting activity in itself. In these cases, imposing a regime of learning new skills maybe more than your VIP can bear.

If there are any mental health problems, or if he is suffering from early-onset Alzheimer's, you may find it's too difficult to 'retrain' your VIP in his daily habits and tasks.

What may seem a simple exercise for an average middle-aged adult can feel like an SAS obstacle course for those already experiencing physical or mental problems. Think about your VIP and assess how quickly you think he can assimilate new ideas and concepts.

5. Social factors

How sociable is your VIP? Does he live alone or within a family? Is he normally gregarious or is he happiest on his own, rarely meeting other people?

The more contact your VIP has with other people, the more likely it is he will rehabilitate quickly. If he is isolated, it can be difficult to modify his behaviour patterns. In all likelihood he will get 'stuck' in his old habits.

Friends and family are more likely to influence the VIP if they are gently nagging him regularly to do different things. I am a great advocate of grandchildren or great-grandchildren jollying along VIPs (if they are available).

If your VIP is naturally quiet and retiring, he may not want to be involved in trying new ideas. He may feel he is being a nuisance. He may feel embarrassed by not being fully in control. If he is more outgoing, he is likely to be happier discussing his MD with other people and therefore coming to terms with it.

6. Where is he on the scale?

It is said that 'we are all on the scale'. This refers to the autistic spectrum disorder scale which is defined as difficulties in social interaction and communication, also by restricted or repetitive patterns of thought and behaviour. With apologies to the autism community, in the field of MD this spectrum is illustrative of problems that are encountered in rehabilitation of the individual.

At the autistic end of the spectrum, the individual wants order in his world and may have difficulty with social interactions, while at the other end of the spectrum people may be quite creative and good communicators.

Both ends of the spectrum have problems with MD. At the autistic end, the individual is devastated by the disruption of his routines, which are precious to him, as his world revolves around them. He wants order within his world, and MD is a major disruptor of his habits and routines. It is very difficult to wean him off his established routines; there is a lot of distress in not being able to live his life along the tram lines that he has carefully constructed over his lifetime.

The other end of the spectrum is much more flexible, and such individuals are likely to be creative in coming up with innovative ideas that can help them out. They are not restricted by their previous behaviour patterns and may even enjoy the challenge presented to them.

However, the long term for either end of the spectrum is not quite what you might expect. The people at the autistic end of the spectrum often do better. Once they have established new techniques, habits and procedures, their natural self-discipline will work to their advantage, locking down new ways of coping. The more creative end of the spectrum may adapt more quickly with processes etc, but their lack of self-discipline may make implementation more frustrating in the long term.

You, and certainly his family, will be well aware of where your VIP is 'on the spectrum'. Just ask, 'how bossy is he?' The more controlling he is, the longer it may take him to adapt, but in the even longer term, he will cope well. While the less bossy may adapt more easily with less stress, in the long term he may find life more frustrating at a low level.

7. Motivation

The examples that illustrate this book are based on real patients I have known, though their stories and names have been slightly altered for reasons of anonymity.

This is the story of a real man.

Ron Saunders's story

Ron was the father of a school friend of mine, Chris. I used to go back to their house after school. Ron was rarely around. He ran a factory making plastic products. Chris's mum Joan would always be there with a selection of dogs, either chihuahuas or miniature whippets. She was a keen breeder of show dogs.

I saw them irregularly over the years when I examined their eyes. The last time I saw Ron he was in his 80s. He came in because he was really struggling with his vision. He had begun developing MD a few years before but now his vision had deteriorated considerably.

He came in with Joan, who stayed in the waiting room while I saw him. Joan had developed dementia and was physically difficult to deal with. She got distressed easily and would cry out loudly about what she thought was happening around her.

Ron was desperate. He didn't want Joan to go into a home while he could look after her, but his vision was very poor due to the MD.

His main worry was that Joan had begun wandering off on her own. Several times she had been out alone, although she didn't know where she was or how to get back home again. The problem for Ron was that if she walked outside, he had no idea where she was. He couldn't recognise her even if she was only a few feet away, unless she called out for him.

Looking after someone with Alzheimer's is exhausting for anyone. With the added burden of MD, it was monumental. Ron was determined to look after Joan. He placed her needs before his own and struggled daily to cope with a woman who now barely knew him, and whom he could no longer see. But he wouldn't desert her.

He had problem solved all his career and he turned that skill to the challenges thrown up by MD. Despite his frustration and fatigue he refused to be cowed and turned his abilities to conquering what was confronting him each day.

It was the most poignant love story I saw in my whole career. The motivation of caring for his wife trumped his own handicap and made him overcome the problems that MD threw at him.

If the individual has strong motivating factors he will fight back against MD. Ron's was the strongest motivating factor I ever came across.

On the flip side, if your VIP has no motivating factors his will to fight will be negligible. This is one of the most individual characteristics of the lot, and probably the most important of all. If your VIP can't see a future ahead of him, he may just give up.

This is where you and this book can alter things. Through education and with a bit of support you can guide your VIP's outlook, giving him a more positive view of his prospects. You probably won't get an epiphany moment, but gradually you can help him by making life easier and tackling his frustrations.

KEY POINTS

The following factors will be a cocktail of influences, either positive or negative, on your VIP's ability to cope with MD:

- **Age of individual at time of visual loss**
- **Severity and speed of onset of the disease**
- **Personality type**
- **Physical/mental conditions apart from vision**
- **Social factors**
- **How controlling he is**
- **Motivation**

The most important thing you can do for your VIP is to give him back hope.

This is the end of the first section of this book on the theory and factors that affect someone with macular disease. With this overview of how and why he is changed by MD, you can begin to influence your VIP back to a life he wants to lead, rather than a life he feels he has to endure.

PART TWO

Start by doing what's necessary; then do what's possible; and suddenly you are doing the impossible

– Francis of Assisi

Here is your dinner, Gran.
Thanks dear.
That's it Gran, use the magnifier to set the timer.
COACH

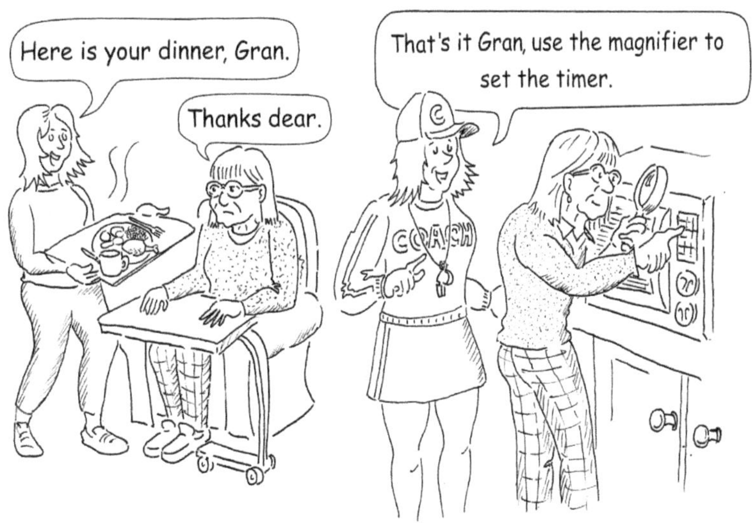

CHAPTER 7

What Your VIP Needs From You As A Coach

You, the 'carer/coach,' are critical to helping a VIP. I cannot stress this enough. You have my admiration and good wishes.

The way we casually use words can influence us. The traditional word for someone with an interest in a VIP is 'carer'. This word was always used unthinkingly, as a useful way of describing a hanger-on in the consulting room.

When I first qualified, the 'carer' was barely allowed into the consulting room with the patient. She was a means to ensure the patient turned up to the appointment. If she muscled her way into the consulting room, she was merely tolerated. Occasionally she had the impudence to ask questions, but generally she was ignored. The hospital was focused first on the disease, then the patient. The carer was a long way down the feeding chain and, with patient confidentiality uppermost, she was rarely addressed.

Working for years with the blind and partially-sighted, my experience and ideas changed. I found I needed to give a lot of information to the patient in a short time. Unfortunately, the patient was unlikely to retain most of the information. Her brain couldn't cope with so much information in one go in such a stressful situation.

I began turning to the 'carer' to make sure the information was understood and that nothing was forgotten when they got home. Gradually I recognised that the most important person in the room was the 'carer'. I could give the information, but the 'carer' was the one who could retain it, and more importantly, implement it.

I also began to question the title 'carer.' There is a subtext to the word that implies that the patient is incapable and is in a permanent state of disability, which is something I don't believe. The visual loss may be permanent, but the inability to cope with the world need only be a temporary state.

This is when I began encouraging the carer to go from a passive role to an active 'coaching' role. The VIP is not ill. She is simply struggling to cope.

The 'carer's' task is to help her VIP 'grow up again.' Initially the role may be that of a traditional 'carer,' when the VIP needs looking after because she can't cope. This is most likely to occur when there has been a sudden loss of vision. This 'caring' should only be a temporary state, though.

You need to switch to the role of a coach after these initial stages. If you are a successful coach you will make yourself redundant as rehabilitation progresses. As a coach, your role is temporary, whereas a carer's role is often permanent.

The role of carer/coach is interesting. It is not normally a position people volunteer for or choose. It tends to come along out of the blue, probably at an inopportune moment.

I doubt you were seeking a long-term role dealing with something you know nothing about and have no prior skills in handling, but by accident – probably of birth – here you are.

You have your own life to lead, and ambitions and desires that have suddenly been ambushed.

The idea of coach rather than carer should be appealing, then, in that it implies that your role should be limited in time rather than a permanent position. Good to know, for both you and the VIP!

To be a coach, you need to have goals in mind and a plan to get your VIP to a specific point.

The plan itself is relatively simple: we need to get your VIP back up Maslow's pyramid. Like the ascent up any mountain, there are different routes, but they all pass through the same levels on their way.

Having read Part One of this book, you should now understand how your VIP is likely to react to her loss of vision. You have to help her through the emotional problems of that loss before you can make real progress with the practical chores and tasks of everyday life.

Part Three of this book will illustrate the main areas that are likely to cause problems for most VIPs. You could just work through these areas one by one, but I suspect most readers are unlikely to do that. Your VIP will have specific, immediate problems that need to be tackled.

Part Three is laid out so as to give a guide to climbing Maslow's pyramid. It is arranged in a particular order to reflect the natural progression in rehabilitating the 'average VIP' back to independence. The point we are aiming for is that your VIP will one day feel strong enough to get out alone, unaided.

Establishing priorities: what tasks need to be tackled?

The first step is to read Chapter 9 to your VIP. This chapter takes the form of a letter from me to help you on your way. When you have read it, it should lead to a conversation with your VIP about her visual loss. Discuss what is bugging her and what she wants to be able to do in the future. This sounds fairly straightforward, but the conversation needs to be done sensitively. This conversation may be casual and easy, or it may end up being emotional and draining.

There are normally two components to the conversation. The first is your VIP's emotional response to all the problems caused by losing her vision. The second component should cover her practical problems – what your VIP needs and wants to do, but is finding difficult.

Both parts of this conversation are important. Often the emotional response is not addressed because both parties are frightened of it. I hope you now understand that the outlook is really not that bad and can be dealt with, but your VIP needs to understand that as well.

The more honest and open the discussion, the better. It should be done in a relaxed way so that you both feel comfortable. If your VIP hasn't expressed her worries and fears before, this is a chance to clear the air. It will help her through the grieving process for the loss of her vision.

You can reassure her that she is not going to lose all sight completely. Although she has lost some vision, she will always keep enough to enable her to get around.

Let your VIP express her regret at not being able to do tasks she has previously loved. Listen carefully to what is being said and the way it is being said. You need to be clear about what she really needs to deal with: her fears and hopes, or practical difficulties.

The temptation is to be judgemental about what your VIP may or may not be able to achieve. Instead, let her blurt out all that is on her mind. She needs to express the worries and fears and grief for what has been lost. Getting that off her chest is a first step in healing.

You can't relieve all her emotional responses in one conversation, of course. These feelings will keep coming out in different ways. Let your VIP talk herself out about her worries. Once she has purged her nightmares you can begin to probe the difficulties she is experiencing.

You know the person you are trying to help. Your goal in coaching is to assist her to the highest level of Maslow's pyramid that she wishes to reach. This process may be relatively limited or it may be a real stretch, but it will be a joint effort between you.

Positive encouragement

It sounds obvious, but your VIP needs lots of positive feedback. You will be applying pressure on her to change behaviour and habits. The difficult bit is to know how much pressure you can apply. Too much or too little can both be counterproductive.

We're back to words again. Try to be positive with any suggestions, or in your shared attempts at doing things differently. Use phrases like:

- *Yes, and... (how about this or that)?*
- *That's a good idea.*
- *Great, let's try it.*
- *How could we make it work?*
- *Let's try it, or test it out.*
- *I like it, that sounds interesting.*

While the discussion is happening, sound enthusiastic and interested. Listen carefully and try to understand what your VIP can and can't cope with. Don't interrupt until she has finished, but build on any of her ideas.

It's easy to kill ideas before they have been fully expressed or explained. Try to avoid phrases like:

- *A good idea, but...*
- *Good in theory, but...*
- *Be practical.*
- *X won't like it.*
- *Costs too much.*
- *Too much hassle.*
- *Too hard to organise.*

Your VIP doesn't want to be talked down to. She already feels vulnerable. People are incredibly sensitive to a patronising tone of voice. They will give up if their antennae register that they are being patronised. I'm lecturing you now, and you will certainly stop reading if you get fed up with me.

Building your VIP's self-esteem with positive feedback feeds the virtuous cycle of progress she needs. We all feel better if someone praises us, and doing things with other people where there is a real connection is what makes us human.

Let her be a toddler

As humans, we are different from most animals. We *dream*. We think about the future, our plans and ambitions. We also think of our past, remembering our triumphs and disasters, the fun times and the difficult times we all experience.

For the VIP, the future and the past will have become something she probably doesn't want to contemplate. There seems to be no useful future for her. The past is that other country that reminds her of what she has lost.

The strange thing about humans is that we often spend little time in the present, which is where stuff really happens.

The present, though, is where a real toddler spends all her time. She hardly has a past and she isn't contemplating her retirement. Play is engrossing. She is fully committed to it. The present moment is all she has.

If you can get your VIP playing, she will be in the moment, and she will enjoy the experience. VIPs often spend far too long in their own heads, thinking of the past or worrying about the future. If you can engage her in the process of brainstorming and playing at changing behaviour she will enjoy it, and forget her troubles while she's at it.

Lower all expectations. You are simply trying things out. Some ideas you come up with may not work at all well. You may discover you can't do something because you need a piece of equipment which is not available. Just bodge the idea along as well as possible to see if it has merit. You don't want to spend a lot of money on equipment that may not be used in the long term. If you have what you think may be good suggestions, slip them in, so your VIP feels she owns the eventual solution.

Try as many different ideas as are practical without exhausting your VIP, all done in a spirit of play rather than deadly seriousness. If you find a winning technique, you may then need to purchase equipment, if it is appropriate to your solution.

The brainstorming process may take time in itself. You may need to let certain problems 'stew' for a bit before returning to them. That is fine. Go about your business. Meanwhile, your minds will have been cultivating solutions in the background.

Go back and have another discussion. Use the question, 'How can this 'goal' be achieved?'

For most of the problems facing your VIP, you will find you get an eventual breakthrough.

When you have your solution, it needs to be practised. Don't let your VIP accept it in theory ('Oh yes, that's a good idea') but not actually do it. You really do have to introduce the solution in real life. The aim is for it to be done with as little thought as possible, in a 'fast thinking' way. Your solution has to be converted to a muscle memory within the brain, a little chunk of action that just happens. This can only work through continual repetition.

Grinding the solution in to the VIP's subconscious so that it becomes a new habit will take a long time. You will need patience. Think of it as like going on a diet. You might want to lose 20 pounds off your waist, but it doesn't happen on the first day of your diet, sadly.

Catherine Cookson's story

You may have heard of the author Catherine Cookson. She wrote romantic family sagas set in the north east of England. Her books sold in their millions.

You are probably unaware that late in life Catherine Cookson lost her sight to MD. She could no longer write. She was devastated by this and went into depression for several months. (This was her working through Kuebler Ross's loss process).

After six months or so, Cookson pulled herself together and did some thinking. She still wanted to be a best-selling author but the act of writing was no longer possible.

Eventually she ended up telling stories to her secretary and husband, who wrote the words down.

Cookson switched from being a writer to a storyteller. The end result was the same – she published books. In fact, she continued to produce bestsellers for eight years after the loss of her sight. But she never wrote another word.

Catherine Cookson's story encapsulates the job of the coach in MD. Cookson knew she wanted to produce books. That was her goal. It was the process of getting to that goal that had to be altered.

Cookson's story takes a few seconds to tell and is obvious when you have heard it, but from her point of view it wouldn't have seemed so simple.

The steps involved:

1. She had to recognise the problem in the first place: how to transfer her thoughts to paper, now that she couldn't write them down?
2. She probably had to acquire recording equipment in some form.
3. Training in use of the equipment was probably necessary, both for her and for the transcribers.
4. She must have had to learn a new technique for writing by dictation rather than writing herself.
5. While implementing the strategy she would have needed support, encouragement and a cheerleader.

I am sure Cookson, her husband and secretary had a glass of champagne when the first book was published. Once the solution was in place, however, it must have been a case of 'move on to the next book and repeat the sequence'.

KEY POINTS

What does the VIP need?

- Let her express her emotional reaction to visual loss.
- Establish what tasks need tackling.
- Use positive encouragement. Build her up. She thinks she is at the bottom of the heap.
- Play. Make it fun. It doesn't have to be dreary.
- Time. You don't need to rush. It can be done s...l...o...w...l...y.

Alone we can do so little;
together we can do so much

– Helen Keller

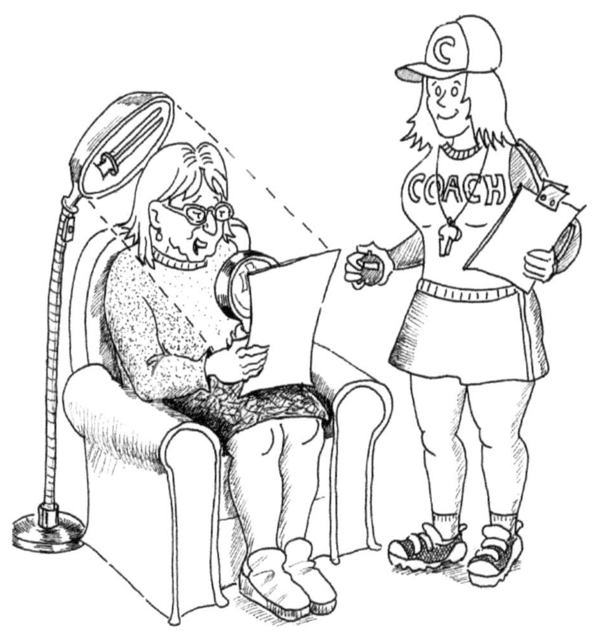

CHAPTER 8

What You Need As A Coach

This chapter is all about you and how to coach someone with MD. We are in danger of just thinking about the VIP and forgetting you. You will be useless to your VIP if you don't also look after yourself.

Like the warning on an aircraft, when the oxygen masks come down: fit your's first, before you fit your child's. You can turn yourself into a martyr by putting your VIP first. That way leads to burnout and disenchantment and backward steps for both of you.

Kevin's story

My father gradually lost his sight as I was growing up. He was and is very independent (and an alpha male type) so it was difficult for him and the family. He insisted that we keep his blindness a secret from everybody, including many members of the family. This perhaps was the hardest part.

I, (like many of the people reading this book) am in the difficult position of being the child and one of the carers of a VIP. This is a tough position. Even when we are adults, our parents still expect to have the final say – which can sometimes cause great conflict and difficulty. Often the carer can't win.

When my brother and I left home my mother had sole responsibility of care. By that time my father had admitted that he was blind (actually he couldn't conceal it any more) and found he was eligible for a guide dog. He also learned Braille at the age of 55 – this is quite an achievement, and is a measure of his "can do" approach to life. My parents were able to retire and have made the most of life. They have adapted well to my father's blindness and have developed all manner of coping strategies. My father says he has never thought: "Why me?", and I asked him once how he coped. His reply (without hesitation): "Because I learn something new every day".

One of the biggest dangers is that the VIP does not permit the carer some free time (time off for good behaviour). We all need some "me time"; otherwise we cannot cope.

In my teenage years there were several painful arguments and threats, when I asked for a bit of time off. (This still hurts because I wasn't being unreasonable). So in the end I found other ways: e.g. taking our dog for longer walks or pretending to have more homework than I did. The other family members also did similar things. At the time,

I was too young to be able to lay down ground rules...but if possible I would urge the VIP and carer to discuss this thorny topic head-on, and agree on some rules.

I remember one occasion when my father had painted a bedroom wall and wanted me to touch up the bits he had missed. I was shocked to find that it was extremely patchy so I needed to repaint the entire wall. I was told off for taking too long, but I couldn't bring myself to explain why. I knew my father was trying desperately to do as much for himself as he could, and the truth would have been devastating, at that time.

I realised at that point that when you are a VIP, you cannot be totally independent. I am sorry but that is a fact, and both carer and VIP need to realise this.

Having said that, it is possible to get a great deal of independence with minimal care – by working together.

In our brainstorming sessions we went with some crazy ideas at times. Sometimes they worked, at other times they didn't, but we then went on to modify our approach.

My father is a very practical man and he wanted to continue DIY projects as much as possible. He learned to do a great deal by feel (putting in screws etc) and my job was to hold the light steady (I learned of the importance of good, properly directed light from a very early age). Sometimes my father was quite reckless, and I wouldn't recommend that.

Often if we were all out he would attempt some project on his own. One day my mother, myself and my brother were out on a shopping trip. My father wanted to repair something outdoors above a ground-floor window so he put a stool on top of a kitchen table (as you do) and proceeded. He then heard a clunk and eventually managed to see the cause of the noise... There on the ground lay one of the table legs! He couldn't maintain his balance indefinitely and eventually took a tumble into the rose bushes!

There were innumerable similar episodes. He fell off scaffolding twice, once into a pile of sand and once on top of me when he mistook my head for my shadow.

And this is the thing; it is OK to laugh at these episodes. In fact it is often very helpful. The development of a sense of humour can save the day.

But my mother is still nervous to leave him on his own because she knows he will get up to mischief!

The carer can gain a lot from this process, too. My dad and I did a lot of brainstorming over the years, and I learned to problem-solve and think very differently. I also learned to make use of my other senses more. I listen very carefully and also use touch a great deal.

There was one event which altered my way of thinking and helped me to cope. I was 15 at the time of the Apollo 13 crisis, and followed the events. After the astronauts were safely returned I saw an interview with Jim Lovell. The interviewer asked the question, "Surely you must have panicked when you looked out the window and saw a massive hole in your spacecraft?"

Jim Lovell replied, "No, I didn't panic, because when you've finished panicking you still have to sort the problem out."

I know that astronauts are selected and trained to be unflappable but I realised that this philosophy has applications in everyday life. Also, the incredible brainstorming and problem-solving that the NASA team had done showed me how human minds can triumph over adversity.

Moreover, you can apply the same reasoning to frustration. VIPs and carers can get very frustrated by the problems caused by sight loss, but getting frustrated only exaggerates and adds to the problems. It is possible to learn to control frustration. (And I should add that it took me quite a long time to get there!). About a month ago we had problems with the drains just before our holiday, and my wife is sure I said, "Houston, we have a problem" when I discovered it.

I would add a footnote to that story. Kevin's father had retinitis pigmentosa, which presents different problems for visual impairment. But the relationship problems encountered are exactly the same.

You have to look after yourself. You need to consider how you can best use your time and energy to help with your VIP's rehabilitation. Your superpowers are limited, and you probably aren't a saint and don't aspire to be one.

This leads on to a serious point about coaching a VIP: it needs to be a team effort. The temptation is to try and do it all yourself, just you and the VIP.

There are problems with the valiant SUPERMAN/WOMAN approach. It takes up a lot of your time, energy and sense of humour. Not only that, but the VIP is likely to get fed up with you constantly hassling them.

Another problem with the solitary coach is that you are unlikely to have all the necessary skills and knowledge to help your VIP. This is not your fault. None of us is skilled in everything.

There are four basic areas with which the VIP is likely to need help:

- Transport
- Technology
- Shopping
- Social life

We will develop these in the following chapters. But it is worth thinking about how these areas can be covered by different people. They fall into categories that will often naturally 'self-select' people who are best-placed to help.

It makes it easier then to get each team member to coach his or her particular area. For one, the VIP gets to meet more people, which itself is good for his self-esteem. You may end up as 'head coach', coordinating activity around your VIP initially, making sure the different areas are covered.

This sounds awfully formal, as if you are going to set up contracts and mission statements with team meetings on a regular basis. You may wish to do that, but in reality, this process is about harnessing local friends, family, neighbours and whoever happens to be around.

You need a selection of people with different skillsets. There are professional people for certain tasks; these will be picked out in the following chapters. Other areas don't need professional qualifications – just enthusiasm.

You will know, yourself, who is best placed to carry out certain tasks. Don't inflict pain on yourself; get others to help. Delegation will make life easier for all. As the saying goes, a problem shared is a problem halved.

Delegating tasks is desirable for several reasons. None of us can do everything well. Do what you do best, and get the others to do what they can, or what they enjoy most.

We all have a certain capacity, physically and mentally. Taking on too many jobs will gradually push up your stress level if you are not careful. Steady work by a team working on different areas will make for faster, easier progress.

It will also reduce the likelihood of guilt, resentment, exhaustion, fatigue, poor health and isolation for you, the coach. You need to be aware of these problems. They can creep up on you if you try to do everything yourself.

At this time, I would like to put in a plug for a book called *The Selfish Pig's Guide to Caring* by Hugh Marriott[5]. It is not about visual loss or blindness. Hugh Marriott's wife contracted multiple sclerosis and the book is his take on how to cope with the caring role. It is a heart-felt account of the trials and tribulations of a carer. The lessons from it are applicable to most carers and it really is worth reading.

An interesting thought on self-help books like this one: most of the people who buy them are avoiding taking action on whatever the book is about. They like the idea of the journey and the end result, but they are more likely to buy another book or course than to actually act.

There is a combination of reasons why this happens.

Often, we stop ourselves from doing something new because it feels too difficult. Insecurity and the possibility of failure can also hold us back.

There are three potential problems:

- Lack of confidence
- Fear of pain
- Laziness

To overcome this resistance, we need to keep the tasks small, and hence less scary. As an added bonus, small tasks give you more opportunities for positive reinforcement.

Reward yourself and your VIP constantly and for almost any sort of accomplishment, big or small. By attaching rewards to desired behaviour, you can increase the likelihood that the behaviour will be repeated.

Develop a reward system that works for you. It should give you energy to attack the next objective. Rewards don't have to be big or even special. They need only be enjoyable and attainable.

---

5 Hugh Marriott. *The Selfish Pig's Guide to Caring*. Piatkus; 1 edition (4 Jun. 2009). ISBN 978-0749929862

The key lies in breaking your objectives into smaller and smaller tasks. Then, when you have found new solutions, find rewards that reinforce behaviour change. (And the little pleasures you get from that are, themselves, gifts.)

Use rewards often and celebrate them. Be optimistic and believe in yourselves. If you go in to any task with a negative mindset and have no confidence, then you doom yourself to failure before you've even started. Try to have faith in your abilities and be optimistic that you will reach your end goal.

Finally finding help

You don't need to reinvent the wheel. There are a lot of people with MD in the UK, let alone the world, so use their collective wisdom. Google is fantastic for advice. Use it whenever you think you have a problem. You won't be the first to have discovered a particular problem; there are lots of interesting solutions out there. You just have to keep searching and using different search phrases. Sometimes the answers may be wild and wacky, but there may be a grain of an idea that works for your VIP from all the pages that are thrown up.

As for local support groups, the Macular Society is number one. www.macularsociety.org

Such groups are often wonderful sources of advice and information. They also supply – as the name suggests – support. The feeling that you are not alone can be extremely important. Local support groups will have been there before you. They can provide invaluable insights and tips about who to talk to and who to avoid, where to go for useful bits of kit, what works, what sounds good but is, in fact, useless.

If you have difficulty finding a support group, search on Google or ask in your local library. You should find several local forums, charities or helplines. Some will be more useful than others, but as a rule of thumb, go to the established charities as a starting point.

Attending a support group gives you the chance to have discussions and general conversation. Often this will provide you with advice or information that you didn't realise was important. Other people are an invaluable resource for you in your role as coach.

There is one final recommendation for this chapter. In association with the RNIB, the charity 'Action for Blind People' runs regular courses. These are an excellent introduction to local help. At present, they offer a beginner's course called 'Finding Your Feet.' These courses are designed for people who have lost vision recently and who still need to 'find their feet,' as the course title says. www.rnib.org.uk/finding-your-feet

The charity also offers general courses that give an overview of the problems associated with losing vision. Such courses are a chance to meet other people in a similar position. This may be the first time you have the opportunity to discuss the common problems.

Consult the internet for information about similar courses near you. They are held all over the UK and usually last one or two days. Although they are aimed at the VIP, I recommend that you attend with him. What you learn will provide a base from which to work. You will get information on what is available locally and how to access it. (I would not recommend attendance if your VIP's visual loss has happened in the past three months, however. He will get more from the course if he is not still in an emotional state due to the loss.)

I hope that as you put the ideas in the following chapters into practice, you will develop new reserves of patience, strength and empathy. It won't always be easy, but you will discover a lot about yourself, and others. Nobody wants to go through these experiences, but you will discover things about yourself and others that may prove invaluable.

You, the coach, are incredibly important to your VIP. I thank you for time, dedication and enthusiasm for getting this far in the book. Well done!

KEY POINTS

- **Create a team for the following different tasks:**
    - **Transport**
    - **Technology**
    - **Shopping**
    - **Social life**
- **To do any of the above, use whatever information tools are available on the internet.**
- **Finally, remember to look after yourself.**

The next chapter is designed to help you kick off your programme of change with newfound information and enthusiasm.

Embrace failure. If something doesn't work, keep going; you have simply crossed off one option on your journey to find a solution that works. It's part of the play process. Don't dwell on it as a failure; see what you can build from it.

To be in hell is to drift; to be in heaven is to steer

– George Bernard Shaw

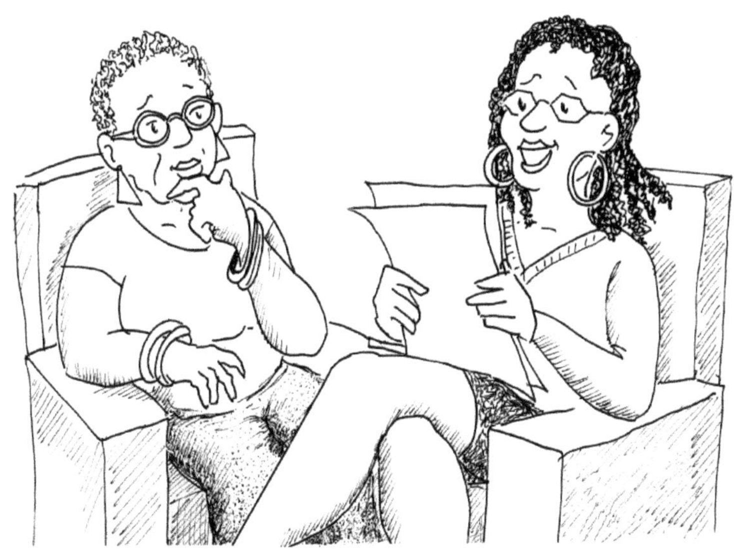

CHAPTER 9

Letter To Your VIP

This chapter is different from all the others in this book. It takes the form of a letter which will explain to your VIP what has happened to her because of MD, and how you are going to work together to improve the situation.

Please read it directly to your VIP. This is so she understands what is happening going forward. It will give you a platform from which you can both work. Having listened to it, I hope your VIP will understand how, together, you can improve her situation.

Otherwise, if you just try telling a family member something, it is likely to be greeted with a lack of respect. 'What do you know about it? Are you suddenly some kind of expert?'

I know it can be galling to hear your VIP listen with attention to an 'expert' telling her something, and then nod agreement, when you have already tried to explain the same thing several times and she wouldn't accept it, but hey, that's families.

Your VIP is going to be more amenable if she hears it from an expert. Just go with it, even if you feel like strangling her as she then explains to you what she has just heard for the 'first' time.

You can personalise this as you go along by inserting your name and hers at appropriate points.

Dear (...VIP's name...),

We have never met and probably never will. Despite this, I know a lot about you. I understand you have lost some of your vision to macular degeneration. I am sorry for you. It is a distressing condition. It causes a lot of problems, which you are painfully aware of.

I have worked with people with macular disease all my working life.

I have asked (...your name...) to read this letter to you so that you can better understand what has happened and how we can try to improve things for you.

Unfortunately, I am not a miracle worker and cannot restore your vision. However, I hope to offer you some insight into your condition and to help you get back to living an enjoyable life.

There are two distinctly different groups of visually impaired people – those who are born blind and those who lose their sight as adults.

You have lived your life with vision. Your habits and lifestyle have been built on being able to see. Losing something you have taken for granted is difficult to deal with.

But if you think of Stevie Wonder or David Blunkett, they never had sight, and yet both have lived full lives.

Their struggle with blindness was much easier than yours, however. They didn't have a problem with lack of sight. It was what they grew up with. As toddlers they learnt how to cope with the world.

You have a much more difficult task. You suddenly have to relearn all those things you previously took for granted. You **can** get back to living a full life, but it will require effort and thought on your part.

You will have been very frightened by your loss of vision, and you may fear that you will lose all vision completely.

What the public thinks of as blind is no light, complete blackness, as when you close your eyes. I have never met anyone who has lost all vision from macular degeneration. It does not happen.

You are detail-blind. You will always be able to get around. You can walk to the shops but when you get there you won't be able see what is going on because of the loss of detail.

In my trade, you have what is known as navigational vision. That lingering fear of blindness that haunts you is just a fear. You will not lose all your sight.

In fact, few people have complete blindness (no light, no movement) as the public understands it. The vast majority of blind people have a certain amount of vision. Hence the term visually impaired, which is what you are.

You know that you can still see quite a lot of things and can get around, but you have difficulty with detail. Because everybody thinks of blindness as having no vision at all you don't regard yourself as blind. Therefore, you may feel guilty about your alleged disability.

You are disabled because of MD, and are therefore entitled to call yourself blind. But you are worried that the general public may think you a fraud, as you can happily wander the streets avoiding children and lampposts. You and they don't believe that you are 'blind'.

Therefore, a better term to use when chatting to members of the public is 'visually impaired', even if you are registered blind. Otherwise there is likely to be a mismatch in understanding. Eye-care professionals will use the term 'blind' in a technical way, which is different from the public's understanding.

Now I want to move on to explain how macular degeneration can affect you, and how to deal with these effects.

But first I am now going to be rude about you. You have probably become a rather grumpy old man/woman recently. The reason for this is that you have gone back to being a 'toddler'.

Let me explain. We have all seen a mother dragging a toddler kicking and screaming out of a supermarket. It is a rite of passage of parenthood. The toddler can't get or do what it wants, so goes into meltdown.

You may have been feeling equally frustrated since losing your vision.

It is highly frustrating, losing vision. You can't do all the things you used to do. You get frustrated with yourself and those around you, and you may become difficult to live with at times.

Occasionally when I have said this to people they tell me honestly that they haven't been grumpy at all. Such people are the exceptions, though. It is perfectly natural to be a bit grumpy. It is because of your own frustration.

A second characteristic of toddlers is that they sleep a lot. They fall asleep at the drop of a hat. You have probably been sleeping a lot more frequently since losing your vision.

The reason is that it is extremely tiring losing vision. You are working very hard. You are probably working harder now than you have for many years.

Why are you working harder? Well, if you have good vision you glance around wherever you are. You recognise people, find objects, and work out people's emotional states by looking at their faces.

When you have poor vision, you can do none of these things. You can make out people's shapes. You have no idea of their emotions because you can't even recognise their faces. Objects in a room barely exist for you until you touch them.

The average person looking around a room uses little brain power. You are using three times as much brain power as they do. You have to use first your normal amount of brain power to look around, and then, because you don't know what you have seen, you have to interrogate this information. You try and get clues to what is around you. You then have to test your hypothesis out. Is that a cup of coffee on the table? Is that my daughter who just entered the room without saying anything?

Your brain is working hard simply to grasp the essentials of what is going on. It is exhausting. You are going to be knackered just getting through the day, which is why you will tend to drop off to sleep more often than you used to.

This exhaustion, because you are using so much brain power for basic functioning, also means you will have little brain energy left over to do anything else. You may find you just can't be bothered to do anything.

It is not uncommon for people with MD to worry that they are getting Alzheimer's disease or are going a bit 'batty'. Stuff they used to be able to do they now give up on.

You are not going batty or getting Alzheimer's. Your brain is frying itself, just trying to get through the day.

Your brain is running slow and using too much power. It is exhausting. You end up frustrated, grumpy and washed-out. Not a great way to be.

Now the good news. There is another characteristic behaviour belonging to toddlers, though it is unlikely you are doing much of it at the moment. Toddlers spend a lot of their time playing. They do all sorts of things for fun and keep repeating them. They love repetition.

As adults, we say they are playing. They are not really playing, though. What they are doing is learning how the world works by experimentation, and by a repetition of skills.

The problem with you is that you are an adult. You know how the world works. You have a lot of experience of it. You no longer feel the need to play.

But, because your visual loss has left you as a toddler, you need to relearn how the world works, and the best way to do that is by playing.

I don't expect you to start crawling around on the floor. As an adult you can use your brain for this. We need to get you to do some experimentation and repetition of tasks.

The problem is that at present you get up in the morning and need to do 153 different things during the day. With poor vision, you are going to stumble around doing 153 things fairly poorly. By the end of the day you collapse frustrated and exhausted.

Next day you get up and repeat the process with the same 153 tasks. It's like Groundhog Day. But we don't want Groundhog Day. It will gradually sap all your energy and vitality.

You are trying to do the tasks the way you have always done them, but your old techniques may no longer be appropriate. Because of your difficulties you will retreat into the 'comfort zone' of known ways and habits. Gritting your teeth, you're carrying on as normal, doing things the way they have always been done, determined not to be beaten.

The problem is that those habits were created by someone who had good vision. They are probably not the best way of doing something when your vision is poor.

What we need to do is find a better way to carry out each task. It's not rocket science.

Each day I want you to concentrate on one particular task and find a different, better way of doing it. Think of this as play. The toddler finds ways of doing things by a process of trial and error, often via random routes. This is what you need to do, but in an adult way.

If you select and solve one problem one day, the next day you will have one task you can do well and 152 things you can't do well. If you keep going, after fifty days you will have solved fifty problems.

Each day, if you find a solution to a problem, it will make life easier for you. It will free up some of those precious brain cells. You will become less tired and have more energy to think about other things.

The more problems you solve, the less grumpy and tired you will become. When your brain is less 'bunged up', you can enjoy life again. More tasks solved, more brain power – it is a virtuous circle.

The trick to an easier life is problem-solving and finding new solutions.

As an example, suppose you've been having problems making a cup of tea. You are worried about making a mess, or scalding yourself with boiling water. That's the problem. How do we solve it?

First of all, you have a cup of tea and settle down. Living with sight loss is all about thinking, really. This exercise is best done with someone else, rather than on your own. You want to generate as many ideas as possible and it is easiest with someone else. (Grandchildren are great for this if they are in the 12-25 age group.)

Have a brainstorming session about ways to make a cup of tea. Any suggestion is allowed. Come up with different ways of getting the water hot enough, then combining it with either tea leaves or tea bags to make a drink in a container you can drink from. This is a back-to-basics exercise.

When you have got a list of suggestions, trot off to the kitchen to try them out. The most important thing is that you have already had a cup of tea, so you don't need or want one while you do the exercise. You're just going to be playing at making tea.

When you've played around with the different ideas, you will find some work and some don't. You are going to waste a few tea bags and some water, but hopefully you will find a new, safe, easy method of making tea.

You might come up with the idea of filling a mug with cold water. Pop the mug in the microwave for a minute or so. When the microwave goes ping, remove the cup, drop a teabag or a spoon of coffee in, slop a bit of milk in, and hey presto – a cup of tea, made safely and with no mess.

This may be the way you always make tea or coffee, or it may never have occurred to you to do it in this way before. But it works. There are a surprisingly large number of ways to make tea, but we tend to use a default method which we never think about, because we have done it so many times before.

This process of relearning the world is, in itself, tiring. This is why you should do it one task at a time, day by day. If you try and solve too many problems at once it won't work, and you will become exhausted and frustrated again.

As macular degeneration doesn't go away, you have quite a while to work on relearning new skills. Take it steadily and you will be able to gnaw away at your day-to-day problems. As the saying goes, 'you can only eat an elephant one bite at a time.'

With the help of (...) reading this book, we can get you back to enjoying life. There is more information in this book to help with the particular areas that are likely to cause most difficulty for someone with poor vision.

There are also suggestions on how to cope. Most of it is about 'why' you are having problems. When you understand the why of the problem, you are half way to solving the problem.

(Take a breather here)

One topic I would like to discuss with you is going out in public.

Since suffering from visual loss, you will have discovered it is now very difficult to recognise people. This is more difficult in public – in the street, for instance – as you won't know who you might run into. You can make out the shape of a person, but the face is a mystery.

You may also have been in a shop where you've had trouble finding what you want. You may have had difficulty paying for a purchase, struggling with coins or notes.

Humans use non-verbal communications a lot. We frown, we smile, we indicate yes or no with looks or gestures. Often, words are not used. Because of your macular degeneration you have lost the key to this non-verbal communication.

If I am standing in a shop and you ask me where the pickled onions are when they are right in front of you, I am likely to think you are taking the mickey. I won't jump to the conclusion you have a visual problem. You look perfectly normal to me. You are walking around with no obvious difficulty.

If you are fidgeting around with money at the checkout you are simply being a pain in the backside as far as most of the public is concerned. People won't jump to the conclusion you are partially-sighted, unless they have some clues.

You have to realise the general public has a stereotypical view of the world. Unless you have a guide dog, or are bumping into things or groping around, you are not going to be judged as 'blind'. The public doesn't understand macular disease.

At a social event, people aren't likely to realise you haven't recognised them. They will probably just think you are a stuck-up old so-and-so because you haven't said hello. This is a particular problem with people who are casual acquaintances. They don't know you have a problem with your sight. Your close family and friends will know your vision is bad, but casual acquaintances or neighbours either won't know or won't remember.

The answer to these problems is a **signal** or **symbol** cane, a white collapsible stick.

A signal cane is now your form of non-verbal communication with the sighted world.

The signal cane makes interactions easier for all concerned.

You don't need a stick for getting around. You can see to negotiate down a street without bumping into things. You don't need to walk along tapping as you go.

The stick, as its name suggests, is a signal or symbol to other people. If you have a symbol cane in hand, it will give them the clue that you can't recognise them. The use of a symbol cane is simple good manners. It is rude not to use one.

You don't need to be waving it around all the time, however. If you're a woman, you are lucky; women tend to carry bags around with them, so you can simply keep the cane folded at the bottom of your bag until you need it. If you think you are getting in trouble, reach into the bag and get it out. In a shop, reach in and use the cane when asking for help. At a social event, have it in your hand as you enter a room.

I particularly wanted to tell you about signal canes because I know there are a lot of issues and resistance around the use of white sticks. People don't like to draw attention to themselves, but not using one is likely to cause more confusion and embarrassment than using one. Signal canes are obtainable from the RNIB website. I really, really would recommend using one in public.

The final point about white signal canes is that people often feel guilty about using one. They think that, as they can wander around OK without any help, they are not 'properly blind' and are not entitled to use a cane.

This is not the case. If you are going to cause confusion around you, or if you feel unsure and apprehensive in public, then use a cane. It will make you, and everyone you come into contact with, feel more comfortable.

(...your name...) reading these words is going to read the rest of the book and will be able help you with lots of ideas in the coming months.

If you take things gently and discuss the problems that are bugging you with (...your name...), together you can make a lot of progress. Just keep problem-solving and remain open to new ideas.

When you have finished listening to this letter, create a list of the jobs that have been causing you problems. Together with (...your name...), you can begin to address them one by one. By thinking about some of your most deeply-ingrained habits and gradually modifying them, bit by bit you can make life easier.

I hope that you found this useful and I wish you well in your efforts to regain your independence.

Yours,
Paul Wallis

The only thing worse than being blind is having sight but no vision

– Helen Keller

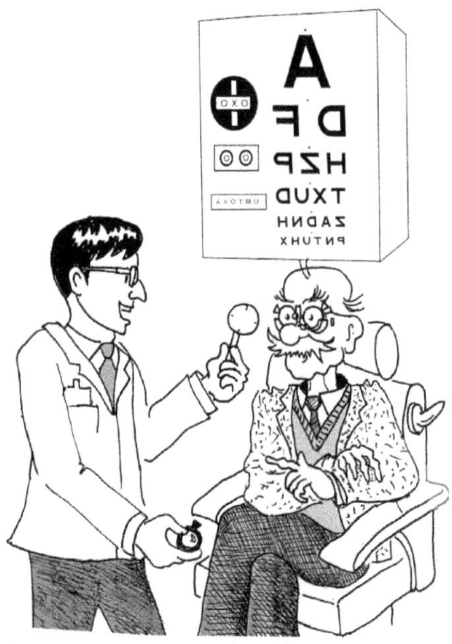

CHAPTER 10

Making The Most Of Existing Vision

Although MD has caused havoc at the macular area, your VIP will still retain some vision. This chapter will deal with optimising that existing vision.

As an optometrist, I would recommend an eye examination by an optometrist. It is an essential starting point. When a VIP has been under the hospital eye service for some time, it may be assumed that the hospital would have sorted out glasses. They often will assume this has been done elsewhere.

The simplest solution is to use your local optometrist. If your VIP has someone he sees regularly, just book an appointment with them. All optometrists can provide you with an accurate prescription for glasses to use for distance vision, television, etc, and a near prescription for close tasks like reading and writing.

Unfortunately, because of the MD, your VIP's vision with these glasses will not be brilliant or a 'miracle cure'. But glasses with an accurate prescription can provide a benchmark from which to work.

I recommend that you or someone else attend the eye examination with your VIP. Sit in on the consultation. You will then have an accurate idea of what his level of vision is. You can also ask questions for both of you to better understand what is going on.

During such examinations the inevitable question is usually raised: 'Can I just have stronger glasses to read with, please?' This sounds like a reasonable request, but it creates a certain amount of confusion.

Distance glasses are designed to let you see an object like a road sign by focusing the light from the road sign exactly on to the retina at the back of the eye. Each eye has its own prescription that does this.

There is no magnification involved in distance glasses. You can't make an object at a distance appear bigger or smaller with a pair of glasses. You would have to use some form of telescopic device to make something appear bigger or smaller. A pair of glasses simply would not fit the bill.

With reading glasses, the situation is slightly different. The lenses are designed to focus the light from an object, such as a book, precisely onto the retina. However, with reading glasses we can choose where the book is held.

We can therefore make glasses 'stronger' for reading, but the price that is paid for this 'strength' is the reading distance. The stronger the glasses are, the closer the book has to be.

The normal, accepted distance for reading is approximately 40-45cm, which is about the distance at which you would hold a book in your lap. This is a comfortable position from which to read a book with normal print and with normal vision.

When vision is too poor to see normal print, font size 12, the easiest thing to do is to bring the book closer. With normal reading glasses, however, bringing the print closer will make it go out of focus.

If you make the glasses 'stronger' what you are doing is bringing the point of focus of the lenses closer than the normal 40-45 cm.

While you are at the optometrist's, you can ask him to illustrate this for you by simulating 'stronger' glasses. If the focus is moved in to 25 centimetres (10 inches) the book will be bigger and easier to see. In the optometrist's chair this may be acceptable because your VIP will be reading from a lightweight piece of card.

At home, however, holding up a large print book at a similar distance would quickly become heavy and tiring. Sheer lack of muscle power would stop your VIP from reading for long periods of time.

The power of the lenses could be further increased so that the working distance is only 10 centimetres. Your VIP would then be literally holding the book at the end of his nose. This reading distance would be extremely tiring for long periods, but some people find it acceptable for certain tasks, like reading invoices or instructions.

The optometrist can give your VIP the opportunity to try these 'stronger' lenses out. The normal reaction is, 'I don't want to read like that!' This is understandable. He is hoping to go back to reading 'normally' with a book in his lap.

Depending on the degree of vision that has been lost, stronger reading glasses may be all that is needed to make reading easier. If stronger glasses don't work for your VIP then it is time to move on to magnifying glasses, but I will deal with those more fully in the next chapter.

Jean's story

Jean was bought in to me by a concerned daughter-in-law. She had lost sight due to MD and could no longer read. She had been living with her family for a couple of years. She watched the telly, but didn't do much else. The hospital had been giving her injections regularly, first in one eye, and now every few weeks in both eyes.

Her last eye examination had been about five years before when she was first diagnosed with MD.

On questioning, Jean admitted she could pick out print if she held the book very close. Having examined her, I discovered that owing to her diabetes and early cataracts, she had become more short-sighted.

With an accurate prescription for glasses I was able to miraculously 'cure' her MD so that she could read again. The injections were holding back any visual loss quite effectively, but her eyes had aged coincidently.

The daughter-in-law was delighted. Her mother could now read the smallest print with ease. I am not quite so sure Jean herself was that delighted, as the disability that got her attention and sympathy had been rather abruptly removed, and she felt a bit of a fraud. She genuinely had a problem, but it wasn't the problem she'd assumed. Needing new glasses is nowhere near as dramatic as going blind.

Other ways of enhancing vision

Tinted lenses

Light is, obviously, what lets us see. But light itself can be a problem for the VIP. Regulating the amount and type of light getting into the eye can make life easier or more difficult.

For various reasons, the individual may be more light-sensitive when outdoors, so some form of tinting of glasses can be helpful. The type of tint and level of tinting will be critical and will be different for each of us.

For most of us, the point of sunglasses is to reduce the amount of light getting into our eyes when lying on a beach on holiday.

When you are shopping in February at your local supermarket, it is a different situation altogether. You are trying to reduce glare, while simultaneously improving contrast and letting as much light into your eye as possible.

There are four factors at work here:

1. The light transmission factor of the lens
2. The colour transmission of the lens
3. Glare reduction
4. UV protection

1. Light transmission. All lenses stop a certain amount of light getting through a lens. A 'clear' spectacle lens only transmits 92% of light through it (a specialist would say this lens has an LTF of 92%), but nevertheless the lens appears clear. If you are in very strong light conditions you can use a 10% LTF. This lens is very dark and would only be used by a normal person in exceptionally bright sunlight.

You can specify the level of transmission that is needed. If a lens is used inside then a 75% LTF lens will take the glare from indoor lighting. However, this lens would not be adequate in full sunlight.

You will need to discuss this with a dispensing optician who can demonstrate the different levels of tinting available. It is a careful balance, involving lowering the light level just to the point where it is useful but not so low as to make the VIP's vision worse.

2. The colour transmission of the lens is also critical, to improve contrast. Essentially, this is the colour of the tint. When you have MD, you can choose a tint to improve vision by selecting within the yellow/amber/orange/brown colour range. This will reduce the amount of light getting into the eye whilst simultaneously increasing the apparent contrast of what you are looking at.

There are various sunshields available for MD. Some people find them invaluable, others are unimpressed, but while you are at the opticians they are certainly worth trying out. Sunshields may be used both indoors and outdoors, but different shields are necessary for each option.

3. Glare reduction. Glare can be reduced significantly by using polarised lenses. This is often more of a problem when your VIP also has cataracts, as these create a lot of glare.

4. UV protection. Finally, incorporating a good UV filter in the glasses will help prevent any more damage to the retina.

Eccentric viewing

There is one final way to use vision better. It is called eccentric viewing. If your VIP has said to you at any point, 'I can see something clearly, then it disappears,' this indicates that he may well retain a useful island of vision – in which case, eccentric viewing is the answer.

This technique can appear to be a bit of a dark art. It is often alluded to in books and on websites. It is quite straightforward, but it is a 'Marmite' option – It either works or it doesn't. It is almost impossible to predict whether it will work from person to person, due to the uniqueness of each individual's sight loss.

The theory is straightforward. When MD attacks the eye, it does so in a random way. Like rust attacking the bodywork of a car, the damage around the macula is patchy. Some bits are destroyed while some are untouched. This can leave 'islands of vision' in a sea of darkness. These 'islands' can be utilised if you know where they are. The art of eccentric viewing is locating these islands and making the most of them.

You may notice some visually impaired people won't look straight at you. David Blunkett in TV interviews always looks well away from his interviewer. This is not because of rudeness or shyness – he is simply trying to see them with an off-centre area of his retina. He is using eccentric viewing.

How to learn eccentric viewing

Get the VIP to sit in front of you, facing you directly from a distance of about 4 to 6 feet. You also need to be sitting down.

Ask him how clear your face is on a scale of 1 to 10 (1 being poor, 10 being good). They may say 3 or 7. This gives you an idea of how clearly he thinks he is seeing when looking straight ahead.

Now hold your left hand to the side of your face and ask him to look at your hand. While he is looking at your hand, ask him how clear your face now is. He has to fix his gaze on your hand, not your face, but he should still be aware of your face to one side.

This exercise is a bit like the trick of trying to pat your head with one hand while rubbing your stomach with the other. The VIP will be trying to watch your hand while simultaneously being aware of your face.

Observe his eyes while doing this exercise. Make sure he is assessing your face without looking away from your hand.

Now repeat the exercise with your hand to the right of your face. Repeat with your hand above your head and then below. Each time the VIP should be looking at your hand but being aware of your face.

Your VIP may say your face looks a bit clearer when he is looking towards the right or the left.

Next, remain sitting opposite him, but hold your hand above your face, your face still visible. Slowly move your hand around your face, like the hand of a clock. Move from the 12 o'clock position via 3 o'clock, 6 o'clock and 9 o'clock before returning to 12 o'clock.

Your hand makes a circuit of your face. All the while, your VIP should be staring at your hand, but being aware of your face.

When you have finished, ask him, 'Was my face clearer when my hand was in any particular position?'

He may say, 'Yes, when I was looking at the 4 o'clock position' (for instance). If and when an area of better vision is located, it can be utilised by your VIP, with a bit of practice.

We are all hardwired to look directly at whatever is of interest. This puts the object's image on our macular area. But if the macula is not working, we need to put the image onto the next-best area. This is eccentric viewing.

The way to make use of eccentric viewing is for your VIP to look directly at whatever he is interested in, then drop the vision to the 4 o'clock position (or wherever the vision is better).

A simple way of practising eccentric vision is while watching television. The sitter, your VIP, is not moving, and the TV is stationary. If the television news is on, there should be a person located centrally on the screen. Get the VIP to stare straight at the presenter, and then to let his eye roam around the periphery of the TV in a spiral, moving out from the centre and around the face. He can then find his 'sweet spot' of vision.

Once your VIP has located the 'sweet spot' he will have a better image of the screen. He then needs to practice looking directly at what he wants to see and then shifting his line of sight to use the sweet spot. Watching TV is a useful way of practising this.

If your VIP doesn't understand the principle of eccentric vision, objects may pop in and out of vision for him, seemingly at random. With eccentric viewing, it will become easier to see and maintain focus on something. Initially it may feel wrong to look away from something in order to see it, but your VIP will learn with practice that by looking in the 'wrong place', he will things see better.

The reason eccentric viewing is a 'Marmite' option is that your VIP's visual loss may not have left him with any islands of better vision. If there is a diffuse loss across the whole eye, eccentric viewing won't help.

If there are any islands of vision, your VIP will probably have started to use them already, even if it is not a conscious practice. Having this process explained gives him 'permission' to look in the wrong direction.

Ellen's story

Ellen came to see me with her son. She had lost vision to MD about a year before, in her left eye. The right eye had been poor for over five years. Ellen lived on her own in a retirement flat. The relationship between the generations was a bit tense; her daughter-in-law was not sympathetic. They had clashed on several occasions, underlying which was the question of just how bad Ellen's vision really was. Her daughter-in-law thought she was just attention-seeking from her son.

Paradoxically it was because Ellen was coping well that the problems arose. She could recognise the family when they arrived, because she had so few visitors she always knew it was them. She could get around the flat and her guests with apparent ease.

The incident that caused all the problems occurred when her granddaughter was playing one afternoon on the floor. She had a little dolls' house with all its assorted furniture and accessories. One of the pieces had rolled away across the floor. Ellen helpfully pointed out where it had gone.

This was the moment when the daughter-in-law decided Ellen was having everyone on with her 'poor' vision. Ellen was watching TV, getting around OK on her own, and now she could see small objects. How could there be anything wrong with her vision?

Ellen had picked up on eccentric viewing and was doing it to make the most of her vision. She was automatically looking away to see things more easily. The toy incident was partly eccentric viewing and partly the movement of the toy as it flew across her line of sight.

When I had examined Ellen's eyes, I explained to them that she was in fact eligible to be registered blind if she wanted to be. This was greeted with surprise and relief by her son, who realised that Ellen's complaints were perfectly legitimate. I also explained how it was that Ellen was able to see small objects out of the corner of her eye if they suddenly moved or caught the light. However, they would 'disappear' when she looked directly at them. This is what was creating confusion in the family.

I also explained why Ellen was no longer looking anybody in the eye. She could see them better by using eccentric fixation, but the sideways look was making her appear uninterested in things and a bit 'shifty' to boot. In fact, Ellen was trying hard to see as well as possible.

The blind registration gave Ellen official permission to be blind. Her family were more understanding once that happened.

Charles Bonnet syndrome

While we are on the subject of vision and its effects, there is a strange phenomenon that can cause a lot of distress if it is not understood.

My old partner at work experienced it with some interest. In low lighting conditions, usually in the late afternoon or early evening, he would 'see' bunny rabbits hopping around the room.

Other people I have talked to have seen faces or brick walls, but often it is some form of animal that appears in the vision. It may be amusing to read this, but it can be very frightening to experience it if you don't understand what is happening.

In these cases, because the macula is damaged but not destroyed, it is transmitting information to the brain, but the image it transmits is mangled. When the information gets to the brain, in an effort to make sense of it the brain decides to 'make something up' – hence the imagery of bunny rabbits or brick walls.

This tends to happen in low lighting conditions when there is less general visual information around, so the brain has freer rein to interpret it how it wants.

This can be very alarming to the VIP and he may be worried about mentioning it. He is already unsure of his own mental state, as we have seen; these 'visions' further convince him he is only one step away from insanity.

It must be stressed to him that this is a purely visual phenomenon, a side effect of the damage to the back of the eye. It is nothing to do with his mental state. It is worth discussing this possibility with him, just in case he has not mentioned it because of worry.

Surgical interventions

There are other means of enhancing vision which are by no means straightforward and which require the skills of an ophthalmic surgeon.

There have been various experimental attempts to implant optical telescopes within the eye. There have also been attempts to implant electronic devices either within the eye or connected to the visual system. These come up fairly regularly in the press as a 'technological breakthrough to cure blindness'.

These options need to be looked at and assessed objectively. Most are experimental and are more a matter of aspiration than reality. They are obviously outside the scope of the DIY help that we are concerned with in this book.

I am not a great fan of these techniques for several reasons:

- There is a danger of damaging the eye further while fitting these devices
- The vision created will be very strange even if the operation is successful
- If the VIP is unhappy with the result, undoing such operations is difficult. It would require another operation, with further risk to the eye.

Due to the hardwiring of our visual system, we have a model within our heads of how the world should look. Fitting a telescopic device within the eye would lead to the brain having great difficulty dealing with a radically different image. The proportions and positioning of objects would seem very different.

Imagine wandering around with a pair of binoculars strapped to your head that you couldn't remove. The world would be clear, but it would be magnified. Trying to walk or pick things up would be very difficult.

The ground would seem very close and objects on a table would appear to be inches away, rather than feet. Your whole perception of distance would be completely alien. You would likely feel seasick just trying to walk around.

If your VIP is interested in this form of treatment, please research it thoroughly. I would obtain two independent opinions before going ahead with surgery.

This is where people with sudden-onset loss are at most risk of jumping in, in search of a 'quick fix.' They may not understand the full implications of what they are doing. But I'm afraid if they are happy to be a guinea pig for research purposes they will be warmly accepted, particularly if they are paying for the privilege.

KEY POINTS

- Get an eye examination. New glasses for TV and reading may be necessary
- Try out tinted lenses to reduce glare and increase contrast
- Assess lighting. More lights and stronger lights are generally better
- Eccentric viewing. Try this out to see if it helps
- Consider new technology within the eye, but recognise that it is experimental

At this point, the average optometrist will have done all he or she can. You may need to move onto a different type of practitioner for more specialist help.

Reading is everything. Reading makes me feel like I've accomplished something, learned something, become a better person. Reading makes me smarter. Reading gives me something to talk about later on. Reading is the unbelievably healthy way my attention deficit disorder medicates itself. Reading is escape, and the opposite of escape; it's a way to make contact with reality after a day of making things up, and it's a way of making contact with someone else's imagination after a day that's all too real. Reading is grist. Reading is bliss.

– Nora Ephron

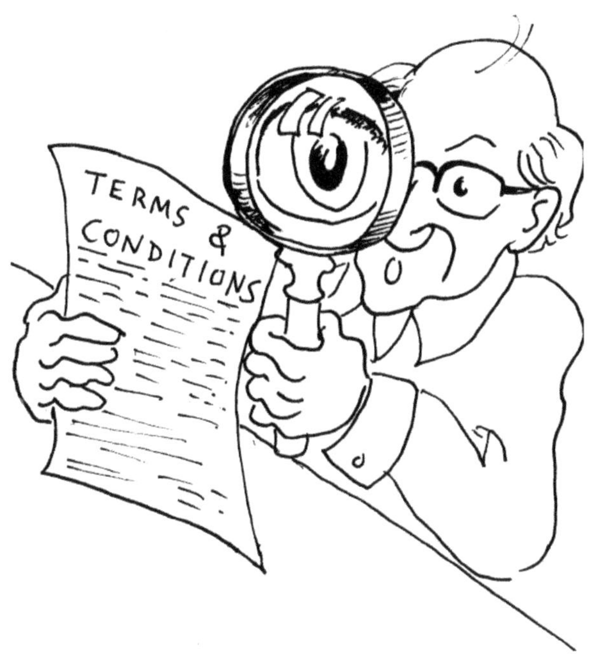

CHAPTER 11

LVA Practitioners

Reading

Having obtained the best possible vision with glasses we now have to step up a gear. This is where my particular career comes into play. I am an LVA, a low visual aids specialist. I see people daily. I will try to obtain the best visual result I can, but I am not a miracle worker. My role is often about framing expectations and understanding what is possible.

What is an LVA specialist?

An LVA specialist is either a dispensing optician or an optometrist who is trained in helping people with poor vision.

The LVA practitioner's main advantage over the average optician/optometrist is the range of devices at her fingertips that she can demonstrate and discuss. Because of her specialisation she will understand the problems and frustrations experienced by VIPs. She will be able to shortcut to solutions that are most likely to help.

LVA specialists can be tricky to find, depending on where you live. To find a practitioner locally, ask your own optician or optometrist. They are almost certain to know where you can find someone, though your nearest LVA may not be local.

Alternatively, ask your hospital eye department. They may provide an LVA service in-house or know of a local provider. Asking the hospital is always a good idea. They may provide more help than you imagine. LVA is an area that is often overlooked in a busy clinic, but a gentle nudge may work wonders when you are seeking information.

The quote at the head of this chapter is from the film *When Harry met Sally*, written by Nora Ephron. Her world revolved around words.

The act of reading is something we take for granted. It takes the average child about three years to master the process of reading fluently and understanding what she is reading. Once she has mastered it, it becomes an everyday activity. However, it is the most significant ability we possess as human beings.

You are staring at a piece of paper or a screen right now and you are thinking my thoughts. Silently, I am communicating with you. We have never met and probably never will, but I am telling you stuff and you are listening to me.

That power of thought transference is extraordinary. It is the essence of being human. When most people think of reading as an activity, they think of reading a book, as you are now. Unfortunately, though, an LVA practitioner is not likely to get your VIP back to reading the latest bonkbuster or Booker-shortlisted novel. Our aim is functional vision.

Your VIP has been through a stroke-like experience. She is struggling with many aspects of life. She may be suffering from a form of post-traumatic stress disorder. She needs time while she rambles back up Maslow's pyramid.

The LVA practitioner will be aiming to get her enough vision to live safely: information from books, labels, instructions on packets, phone numbers, shopping lists, tickets, timetables, emails, prices, a tape measure – the basics of life.

Functional reading covers questions like, *How do you cook this microwave meal? Am I about to poison myself with these pills? How much does this pair of socks cost?* We need such information to survive.

There is one further aspect of reading that an LVA may be able to help with. There is usually an assumption that reading is done at a close distance and most of it is, but not all. We also read at a distance: street signs, notices across a room, rail and bus information.

The number one tool used by an LVA practitioner is magnification. There are various ways of using it:

1. Make the object bigger
2. Bring the object nearer to you
3. Use a magnifying glass
4. Use an electronic aid
5. Use a telescopic device

Distance reading is important, but tends to be a secondary problem. The VIP has to be outside and on her own before it becomes an issue.

Near reading is regarded as 'proper' reading and is the most important hurdle, so we will deal with that first.

Reading at near distances

When using magnification to enhance the VIP's vision, the first step is to work out what font size print she can actually see at present with her normal glasses.

To give you an idea of size of print in common use, the font size of newspapers is somewhere between N10-N12 in the body of the paper,

The classified ads may go down to N6.

With MD, the fall in vision is likely to mean the VIP can only read print of N18 (this size of print), with anything smaller being unreadable.

It may be she can only read

N60, or bigger.

The LVA specialist will be trying to get her back to reading N8.

This line of print is N10. It may seem excessive getting her to be able to read N8, given that people rarely need to do so.

The reason LVAs try to get VIPs to N8 is that if a VIP can just pick it out, she should be able to read N12 relatively fluently. She then has a buffer, so that she is not straining too hard to pick out each letter of a word, which would be very tiring.

Working out the magnification needed is not rocket science. If you want someone to read N8 when she can only read N72, she will need 9x magnification. If she can read N18, then she needs 2.25x magnification to get to N8.

This appears to be a straightforward process. However, there is a certain art to it due to the unique nature of each individual's vision loss. Sometimes more magnification is necessary.

If the optometrist has given a 'typical' reading glass prescription of 3 dioptres, the LVA practitioner can demonstrate a 'stronger' pair of glasses with a higher power and with the corresponding shorter working distance. This may be acceptable as a solution, as we saw in the last chapter.

Assuming a higher-power pair of reading glasses is not adequate, the LVA practitioner would move on to a magnifying glass.

Magnifying glasses

The majority of VIPs want a 'big strong magnifier'. What they are asking for is a magnifier that will let them see the whole of the page, while also giving them the magnification to pick out each word clearly. They want a 'big strong magnifier' to let them carry on reading the way they used to.

Unfortunately, this is where we run into the immutable laws of physics. A big magnifier is a weak magnifier and a strong magnifier is a small magnifier. The maxim 'the bigger the better' does not apply to magnifiers.

A big magnifier is weak. A 3x magnifier will give a large field of view. You can see 8-9 words at a time, because it is 80-100 mm wide.

A 10x magnifier is strong but small, only about 30mm wide. It will only let you see 2-3 words at a time.

The worse the visual loss, the higher the magnification needed, and stronger magnifiers get progressively smaller. This is the dilemma for LVA practitioners. They have to give the lowest magnification possible for the largest field of view. It is a difficult compromise: the weaker the magnifier the easier it is to scan the page, while the stronger the magnifier the easier it is to pick out the words.

There are three types of construction for magnifiers.

- The simple, handheld lens on a handle version. You have to constantly hold the lens at the right distance from the book with this type of magnifying glass. You are forever wobbling your hand or the book around to maintain focus.
- The second version has the same stick construction, but with the addition of an inbuilt light. The best lights are LED bulbs, as the light tends to be brighter and they use less battery power. The light makes a big difference because the magnifier itself will obstruct natural light getting to the page. There are a few mains-powered magnifiers available, which never run out of batteries, but which do tie you to a plug socket.

- The third type is a lit magnifier with an inbuilt stand. The VIP can rest the stand on the paper at the right distance to focus automatically. This means she is not hovering her hand over the page trying to maintain focusing distance.

If most reading is done at home, then the third type – the stand magnifier with a light – is normally the best option. The simple 'stick' hand magnifier is useful if the VIP is out in public, or just pottering about and wanting to check something quickly. The handheld variety can be carried easily in a pocket, while the stand illuminated magnifier is probably too bulky if your VIP wishes to read on the move.

There are many different magnifiers in all sorts of sizes, shapes and weights. Some are family heirlooms and some come from Christmas crackers. People will find their own favourite.

The critical components of magnifiers are:

1. Power of magnification
2. Size – field of view
3. Illumination/non-illumination
4. Stand – ease of use for long periods
5. Weight – critical if the VIP is arthritic (the lighter the better)
6. Colour – the magnifier itself should be easily visible

Having a strong lens (high dioptre lens) will give more magnification but not necessarily a good-quality image. If it is a cheap magnifier the design won't minimise aberrations and distortions. The quality of the image may be poor in the periphery of the lens.

A good-quality magnifier has an aspheric design. Instead of a simple spherical curved surface, the surface has been smoothed off at the edges. This stops distortion such as coloured fringes around objects. It also eliminates the 'pin cushion' effect at the edge of the lens. Creating these complex curves is expensive but makes the magnifier more comfortable to use. A cheap magnifier is more likely to induce headaches.

You may come across advertisements in the weekend newspapers selling whole page magnifiers. This sound perfect, offering your VIP the chance to see the whole page with magnification. Unfortunately, they don't work. If you are happy to waste a few pounds feel free to buy one!

Their construction is very lightweight, which is great as they are easy to hold for long periods. However, there is a lot of distortion created by the Fresnel lens design. The main problem, though, is their lack of sufficient magnification to make print big enough to see.

Finding the right magnifier is a case of sorting through the various factors above to seek the best possible combinations of characteristics, with sufficient magnification being the overriding factor. The LVA practitioner should be able to demonstrate a variety of different examples for different purposes.

As a general rule, most people need at least two magnifiers: a larger, more robust magnifier for use in a favourite armchair (or wherever they do most of their reading), and a second magnifier for use while out and about. The second should fit in a purse or pocket, where it can be quickly whipped out to check prices, tickets, food packets etc.

Once you have these two basic magnifiers, your VIP may collect others that are used for various jobs. She may keep magnifiers scattered around the home wherever she does relevant activities, which saves having to carry them around.

How do you use a magnifier? This sounds like teaching you to suck eggs, but a little knowledge is always helpful.

- When reading with a magnifier, the natural way to use it is to hold the paper in your hand in your normal reading position. You then hold the magnifier over the page and look at the print through the magnifier. This is what I call the 'Sherlock Holmes method.' But it is wrong.
- The best way to use a magnifier is to bring the magnifier right up to your eye as if it were a spectacle lens. You then bring the paper you want to read right up towards

the magnifier. Depending on the magnifier, this will be far closer than you would ever normally look at something.

- The reason for using this method is that the print will be far easier to see at this distance, plus the field of view will be much bigger, making reading easier. The more words you can see at a time the easier it is to read. You will have more context for them, as opposed to the words seeming isolated and random.
- This next point also seems counterintuitive – but again, it really is helpful if you can persuade your VIP to do it. When we read we hold a book or newspaper in our hands and scan our eyes across it. (This point is so obvious that I have to draw your attention to it.) When using a magnifier, the precise opposite is ultimately better. You hold the magnifier virtually clamped to your eye, then slide the book or newspaper across the magnifier. Initially this 'feels wrong'. It has to be consciously practised until it becomes a habit. Once that happens, though, it will speed up the rate of reading.
- Reading glasses should be worn when using a stand magnifier that is rested directly on the page. The magnifier is designed to be used with the vision corrected by glasses, otherwise the image will be slightly out of focus.

A hand magnifier is the standard way of improving reading ability for printed matter. However, some VIPs will want a way of reading that involves holding something at a normal reading distance and then having it 'magnified'. This is possible, but we are now moving away from a simple single lensed magnifier. This form of magnification requires a type of telescope.

Short distance telescopic systems can be useful in certain situations. But first let me explain a little about the world of telescopes.

Reading at a distance

Reading at distance tends to be neglected, because close reading is the most obvious problem for your VIP. Distance reading is a problem that often lurks undiscussed. If the VIP has lost confidence and self-esteem, the prospect of venturing outside alone becomes a major challenge.

It can be a Catch-22 situation. The VIP won't go out because she can't see. To try and break that cycle, a device to let her see at distance can begin to restore confidence.

To assist with better vision for train information boards and bus numbers, a telescopic aid held up to the eye may do the trick. The LVA practitioner can help find a suitable telescope, but it will not be the first problem she will tackle. Close reading is the number one priority.

There are lots of telescopes available for use by VIPs, but they are not the Jack Sparrow, leather-bound variety. You can spot the problem: a pirate's telescope is big and long, and therefore not much use in your local high street or for watching television. The pirate telescope uses an 'astronomical' system of lenses to create its magnification, and it also turns the image upside down.

A small, discreet telescope is what is needed. This type of telescope lets you view an object at distance when you can't get closer to it, ideal for things like signposts or shop signs.

There are two different system of lenses used to create a telescope that gives the magnification needed without making the telescope too big.

I don't want to tie you up with the mechanics of telescopes, but the two systems are called Galilean and Keplerian. They both provide magnification, but because of the way they do it they are very different. Both have advantages and disadvantages, which is why I will spend a little time on them. Please bear with me.

The Galilean system is a simple, two lens set-up that is relatively light in weight. Galilean telescopes can be either near-focused or distance-focused; because of the simplicity of design and the light weight, they can be made into spectacle-mounted devices for reading or distance viewing (generally used for TV), but their magnification is not that high.

Keplerian telescopes are what most people think of as standard binoculars. They are heavy, due to an optical design which is more complicated than the Galilean. This design requires the use of prisms to ensure the image you are looking at is the right way up. The prisms, unfortunately, push the weight up quite considerably. The weight means Keplerian telescopes have to be handheld rather than spectacle- mounted. However, the magnification and clarity of image is very good.

Although people think of telescopes as being for long distances, the Keplerian version can also be used for close distances. You could use one for reading, by focusing on a book at a normal reading distance of 40-45 cm, or 18 inches.

There are problems with using telescopes. The first is that any small head or hand movement is greatly magnified. When looking through the telescope the world will swing and sway quite alarmingly despite efforts to keep it steady. This can cause motion sickness in some people if used for any length of time. And this problem is compounded if the thing you are trying to see is itself moving.

Telescopes are best used for watching an object which is static when the VIP is also static (i.e. in a chair). They also work well where the VIP just wants to check information quickly.

The second problem is that a telescope is designed for use with just one eye, though you can use a double system for both eyes, which works well for distance objects (i.e. binoculars).

Near tasks with a telescope

If your VIP wants to use a binocular telescope for near tasks like reading, please be aware of some potential problems. The two telescopes have to be set up so that they are converging on a particular point – in the case of reading, the words on the page.

When you read a book normally, you point both eyes at the book. The eyes swing in to look at it. If you hold the book closer, the eyes have to 'turn in' more, the closer the book is to you.

A two-lens telescope system has to have both lenses aimed at the reading distance point – generally, a standard distance of 33 centimetres. If the print your VIP is viewing is at any other distance, she will get double vision.

There is very little tolerance in the focusing distance. If the VIP moves her head a couple of centimetres back or forwards, instantly she will get double vision. She will need rock-solid positioning, which is very difficult to sustain for long periods of time. Having said that, some people do like to use a binocular telescope for reading because they can maintain an almost-normal reading position.

Examples of magnifiers and telescopes

Pocket magnifiers: 1710-14: Pocket Hand-Held Magnifier Eschenbach

Stand illuminated magnifier: 1580-63: Eschenbach

TV and near telescopes: binocular low power Coil 4090/02 and 4090/03

Monocular 8.25x 8114 magnification from Coloptics (e.g. for distance viewing of bus numbers)

The above devices, or similar, are the bread and butter of an LVA practitioner's life. They provide the basics. But there are many and varied solutions which the LVA practitioner can help with. Who wants to live on bread and butter all the time?

With the LVA practitioner's advice and expertise, you can try different solutions and see what works for your VIP. It all depends on what she wants or needs to do. You should be able to try out different devices or discuss the pros and cons of other ideas.

There is now a crossover between optical devices and electronic devices to help VIPs, as the digital revolution has reached into the world of the blind. This creates problems for LVA practitioners, as there are numerous new devices advertised and available.

It is difficult to keep up with the supply, and impossible to stock many devices for people to try due to their cost.

The LVA practitioner will be able to give impartial advice on different systems with an understanding of their principles, with their inherent advantages and disadvantages. This means you won't have to deal with a salesmen keen to push a particular system.

LVA practitioners are some of the few people you will come across who understand the problems facing your VIP. Their advice on coping and local knowledge should be exploited as much as possible. They can give invaluable tips on how to deal with life with visual loss.

A final point: blind people often read braille. Therefore, some think that if you go blind, you must learn braille.

Please **don't even consider this for a VIP who has recently lost sight. Her brain is far too overloaded to cope with braille. After two to three years in rare cases it is a possibility, although braille is mostly learnt by youngsters who have either never had vision or who lost it early in life.**

KEY POINTS

- Find an LVA practitioner and pick her brains
- Get two magnifiers, one for reading in a chair and one to carry around in the pocket
- Think about a small telescope for distance viewing

Getting information off the internet is like taking a drink from a fire hydrant

– Mitchell Kapoor

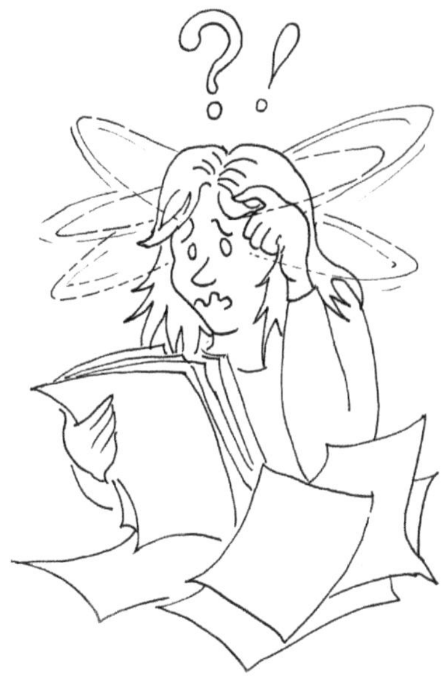

CHAPTER 12

Benefits And Charities

This is a bit of a smorgasbord of a chapter. I apologise that it's a bit lumpy. Think of it as like building a house: the foundations aren't exciting, but they are essential to hold the house up.

Benefits and organisations exist to aid your VIP back up Maslow's pyramid. You can build on their help. They will be your VIP's foundation blocks.

It is useful to get an idea of what is available, and from whom, before you start out. This chapter is a bit of an overview.

There are often significant financial resources available for your VIP, or even for you. Relieving pressure with a bit of money can make coping easier, because vision loss often brings extra costs to a household.

VIPs can sometimes be like the man sitting on the top of his house, surrounded by a flood. A chap comes along and offers him a ride in his boat. The man refuses, saying, 'God will save me'. Then a guy comes along with a helicopter and tries to pick him up. Again, 'God will save me' Eventually a voice booms out from the skies, 'I've sent you a boat and helicopter, what more do you want?'

In Neverland a fairy will alight on your shoulder and whisper information in your ear whenever you need it.

Unfortunately, this is the real world. The temptation might be to wait for help to arrive without asking for it, assuming the world is waiting to deliver whatever it is you need. As we are not in Neverland, though, you'll need to go out and hustle a bit. It is virtually impossible for a VIP to do this for himself. But this is where you can really help him, by finding information and sorting things out on his behalf.

Your local eye clinic will have all sorts of information, but I'm afraid this can be like getting blood out of a stone, depending on where you live. As I have said, you will wait in vain for the NHS to give you guidance and advice. They are there for the disease process alone, but they do have the information available, if you can get it out of them.

Your VIP's hospital may have a counselling service in place for people who have been registered blind or partially sighted – in which case, this may automatically kick in and a referral will happen. In my experience, though, this service is often not available, or else it is administered in a rather random fashion.

The eye clinic may have an ECLO (Eye Clinic Liaison Officer). See the RNIB website for more information (http://www.rnib.org.uk/ecloinformation), although the RNIB itself says that 92% of people are not offered this option following loss of vision. Alternatively, they may have a low vision aid service, the LVA clinic. Ask at the reception desk or speak to the sister on duty in the outpatient clinic about whether they have an ECLO or LVA clinic/service.

After you've exhausted your options at the hospital, there are two main sources of further help. The first is your local county or unitary authority council. They have a statutory duty to help via Social Services.

The second option is one of the 700 charities for blind and visual problems around the country. Neither will come looking for you, however. You have to go looking for them.

The most important resources to access are the state ones. All visually impaired people are entitled to this help.

Even getting access to these resources can be time-consuming and confusing. My best advice is to tackle them one by one. You are about to enter what may feel a bit like a maze with dead ends, false trails and paths that seem to end in mirrors.

Keep your eyes and ears open to all possibilities. You may start off on the trail of one thing but discover something completely different, something that is of greater use in the end. As a rule of thumb, you will get what you need – but it may not be from the source you expected it, or what you thought you wanted.

Let's deal with state benefits first. This information is obviously subject to change.

There are a number of concessions your VIP may be entitled to because of age or sight loss, or both. Skim this lot rapidly to pick out what you think is appropriate.

- Help with NHS costs such as the cost of glasses, eye examinations and prescriptions. http://www.rnib.org.uk/information-everyday-living-benefits-and-concessions-concessions/help-nhs-costs
- You can get a free TV licence if you or someone you live with is 75 or over. And if your VIP is not yet 75, he can still get a 50% reduction in the price of his TV Licence if he is registered blind (severely sight impaired).

- Your VIP's partner (or whoever cares for him) may be able to get extra benefits. Find out more about benefits for carers. http://www.rnib.org.uk/information-everyday-living-benefits-and-concessions-benefits-families-and-carers/benefits-carers
- Consider a Blue Badge that allows any vehicle the VIP is travelling in to make use of disabled car parking spaces. http://www.rnib.org.uk/information-everyday-living-benefits-and-concessions-concessions/leisure-and-travel-concessions
- Blind Person's Allowance to reduce his tax bill (it can also be transferred to a spouse). https://www.gov.uk/blind-persons-allowance
- Free postage using the Articles for the Blind scheme. http://www.rnib.org.uk/information-everyday-living-benefits-and-concessions-concessions/free-postal-service-articles-blind
- You could make use of a free directory enquiries service. http://www.rnib.org.uk/information-everyday-living-benefits-and-concessions-concessions/free-directory-enquiries-195
- There are a range of leisure and travel concessions that can help your VIP get out and about for less. http://www.rnib.org.uk/information-everyday-living-benefits-and-concessions-concessions/leisure-and-travel-concessions

Attendance Allowance

If your VIP is aged 65 or over and needs help with personal care, or help to make sure that he is safe, he could be entitled to Attendance Allowance.

Does the VIP qualify for Attendance Allowance?

The VIP may qualify for Attendance Allowance if he is aged 65 or over and needs help to do things like choosing clothes, reading and replying to mail, walking around safely and taking part in social activities.

- Attendance Allowance is not a means-tested benefit, so it doesn't matter how much other income or savings your VIP has.
- Your VIP can get Attendance Allowance even if he lives alone and doesn't have anyone looking after him; it is his need for the help that is important.
- He can spend any Attendance Allowance he receives however he likes. It can be paid on top of other benefits and may even increase the amount of other benefits he gets.
- If he already gets Disability Living Allowance or Personal Independence Payment, however, he cannot get Attendance Allowance as well. http://www.rnib.org.uk/information-everyday-living-benefits-and-concessions-benefits-people-working-age/personal

Does the VIP have to be registered blind or partially sighted to receive Attendance Allowance?

No, he does not have to be registered as blind (severely sight impaired) or partially sighted (sight impaired) to claim Attendance Allowance. It is how his sight affects his daily living that counts. Registration can provide evidence of how serious his sight problem is. However, you can provide alternative evidence about his sight problem, such as a letter from your consultant or GP.

If your VIP's sight problem is making life difficult, it is worth thinking about getting registered (http://www.rnib.org.uk/eye-health/registering-your-sight-loss). This helps to make sure he doesn't miss out on other help he can get.

How much is Attendance Allowance worth?

If his claim for Attendance Allowance is successful, he will receive one of two weekly rates, depending on how much care he needs:

- a low rate of £55.10
- a high rate of £82.30.

The DWP (Department for Work and Pensions) will take into consideration the care your VIP needs during the day, during the night, and how often he needs that care. There is a factsheet to explain this called **'How to claim Attendance Allowance.'** Use the GOV.UK website for further information.

Pension Credit

Pension Credit is a benefit for anyone who has reached the qualifying age and has a relatively low income. Your VIP may get it even if he has some savings and modest retirement income. It can be paid on top of his state retirement pension.

Pension Credit is made up of two parts, each of which have a different qualifying age:

1. Guarantee Credit has a qualifying age which rises with the minimum State Pension age for women.
2. Savings Credit is for people aged 65 or over.

Your VIP could qualify for both parts, and may even receive an additional amount because of his sight loss.

How do I apply for Pension Credit for my VIP?

Call the Pension Service. Your VIP can also apply for help with rent and council tax, at the same time as applying for Pension Credit. You will need:

- The VIP's National Insurance number
- Information about his income
- Details of any savings and investments (but only savings over £10,000 will affect the calculation for Pension Credit)

Pension Credit can be backdated for up to three months as long as your VIP qualified during that period.

If your VIP is on a low income, there is financial help out there to help him buy the items he needs to assist him in his daily life.

The above details were correct when I wrote them but are probably out of date already. The best port of call for the latest information is the RNIB website (http://www.rnib.org.uk/benefits-and-support).

Guarantee Credit

This is the part of Pension Credit that guarantees a minimum level of income. Should your VIP qualify, the standard minimum he is guaranteed is:

- £151.20 if he is single.
- £230.85 if he has a partner.

To qualify, he must be at the qualifying age and his weekly income (including income from savings) must usually be less than the above amounts.

He may still be able to qualify for Pension Credit if his weekly income is over the above amounts. This may be possible if he qualifies for an additional amount for severe disability or for being a carer, or if he has eligible housing costs such as mortgage interest. The additional amounts often apply to blind and partially sighted people.

If he is entitled to Guarantee Credit, he will also qualify for Housing Benefit or Council Tax Support, regardless of the level of his savings. If he receives Savings Credit only, he will have to make a separate application for Housing Benefit or Council Tax Support.

Your VIP's claim for Housing Benefit and Council Tax Support can be backdated for up to three months, as long as he qualified during that period.

Savings Credit

The Savings Credit is for people aged 65 or over who have modest savings and capital or retirement income. It does not matter if they have a partner who is under 60. This credit provides extra money each week of up to:

- £14.82 if they are single.
- £17.43 if they have a partner.

To be able to get the Savings Pension Credit your VIP must have qualifying income above the 'savings credit threshold' of:

- £126.50 if he is single
- £201.80 if he is in a couple.

Additional amounts for severe disability and for carers

Your VIP may also be entitled to an extra amount for severe disability:

- £61.85 a week if he is single, or for a couple when only one person qualifies
- £123.70 a week for a couple if both qualify.

You and your partner can also get an extra amount for being a carer. You can get this Carer's Premium either because you get Carer's Allowance or because you could get it but aren't paid it because of your state pension. The Carer's Premium is worth £34.60 a week.

Other state help

Approach your local council for help. Your local Social Services may be able to give free equipment and rehabilitation training for daily life. This is a statutory duty. They have to provide it. Often this falls under the remit of the 'Sight and Hearing' team. A lot of these teams have now been subcontracted out to private firms, but they are still council-directed.

Your VIP doesn't need to be registered blind or partially sighted to be eligible for this service. Ask your GP or optometrist to refer him if they don't allow self-referrals.

Benefits for families and carers

Here's a bit more about the benefits you could claim if you are caring for someone with sight loss, or if you are blind or partially sighted yourself and caring for someone.

Disability Living Allowance (DLA)

If you are the parent or guardian of a blind or partially sighted child aged up to 15 then you could be entitled to claim Disability Living Allowance (DLA) on his behalf. DLA is a benefit aimed at helping you meet the extra costs associated with a disability. http://www.rnib.org.uk/information-everyday-living-benefits-and-concessions-benefits-families-and-carers/disability-living

Benefits for carers

See if you could be eligible to receive Carer's Allowance and earn National Insurance credits for looking after someone by reading the RNIB's benefits for carers page. http://www.rnib.org.uk/information-everyday-living-benefits-and-concessions-benefits-families-and-carers/benefits-carers

Carer's Allowance is the main benefit to claim if you are looking after another person. It is not means-tested and does not depend on National Insurance contributions.

To claim Carer's Allowance you must:

- be 16 or over
- not earn more than £110 a week after deductions
- not be in full-time education
- spend at least 35 hours a week looking after a person who receives one of the following benefits:
    - middle or higher rate Disability Living Allowance care component
    - Attendance Allowance (any rate)
    - the daily living component of Personal Independence Payment (either rate)
    - Constant Attendance Allowance

Important: if the person you are looking after receives a means-tested benefit and his benefit includes the severe disability premium, please seek advice before claiming Carer's Allowance, as his benefit may be reduced if you start getting Carer's Allowance.

Carer's Allowance can be backdated for up to three months on request.

How much Carer's Allowance will I get?

The basic rate is £62.10 a week. This is taxable. If you already receive means-tested benefits such as Income Support, you will not be financially worse off by claiming Carer's Allowance.

If you receive a State Retirement Pension, you may not be paid any Carer's Allowance as these benefits overlap.

Can I receive Carer's Allowance at the same time as other benefits?

You cannot normally be paid Carer's Allowance if you receive contribution-based Employment and Support Allowance (ESA), Incapacity Benefit, State Pension or certain bereavement benefits at the same time. However, it may still be worthwhile claiming Carer's Allowance if you get a means-tested benefit such as Income Support to establish 'underlying entitlement' to Carer's Allowance.

This underlying entitlement means you may be able to get an increased amount for means-tested benefits such as Income Support, income-related ESA, Pension Credit or Housing Benefit. The increase is called the carer premium, or the 'additional amount for carers' in Pension Credit. It is worth up to £34.60 a week.

Carer's Credit

Carer's Credit is a weekly National Insurance credit. Although it is not a benefit payment, I recommend that you apply for it as it helps carers to build up their qualifying years for the basic state pension.

You will qualify for Carer's Credit if you care for someone for 20 or more hours a week and one of the following two situations applies to you:

- the person(s) you care for receives the middle or higher care component of Disability Living Allowance, either rate of Attendance Allowance, Constant Attendance Allowance, or the daily living component of Personal Independence Payment
- or a Health or Social Care Professional has certified the person(s) you care for needs the level of care you provide.

Universal Credit

The Government is replacing a number of means-tested benefits that you and your family may receive with Universal Credit. Your VIP may be entitled to a PIP, a personal independence plan payment. Find out more about what the introduction of Universal Credit could mean for you and your VIP here: http://www.rnib.org.uk/information-everyday-living-benefits-and-concessions-benefits-people-working-age/universal-credit

The above covers most of the state benefits. While investigating these locally you may well pick up on local schemes, charities, organisations etc.

Alf's story

Alf and his wife had lived just outside their village all their lives. He was a forester. He enjoyed fiddling with a classic Fordson tractor and taking it to local agricultural shows.

He developed diabetes, and, shortly afterwards, MD. His vision dropped fairly quickly. He was struggling when he came to see me and confessed that the couple weren't coping well financially as he had given up work. Until then he had only been going in a couple of days a week, but that extra money had been essential for them.

I suggested talking to Social Services, not an organisation Alf knew anything about. He had never crossed its threshold in his life.

Next time I saw him he was delighted. He had got a PIP and his wife now received an Attendance Allowance. This funding made a big difference to them. It meant Alf could pay his son-in-law petrol money and they could still go off with their tractor to shows, which now gave him free entry, he told me with a chuckle.

Happy as Larry, he could chew over the advantages and disadvantages of different diesel engines with his mates, most of whom were unaware of his vision problems. Alf had also discovered several ham radio organisations for the blind. He had been an amateur radio user since his teens.

Alf now probably knows more blind people than I do and picks up all kinds of tips and tricks – and not just about radios, either.

Charities for the blind

The RNIB (Royal National Institute for the Blind) and the Macular Society are the two obvious charities you may wish to contact.

They are a goldmine of current information. Although they are not the easiest of reads, please go to the pages mentioned below. You will pick up wonderful tips and help.

The RNIB has several further pages of particular interest:

- http://www.rnib.org.uk/practical-help
- http://www.rnib.org.uk/our-services
- https://www.rnib.org.uk/talking-books-service
- http://shop.rnib.org.uk/

The Macular Society also has some good stuff:

- https://www.macularsociety.org/local-support-groups
- https://www.macularsociety.org/counselling

Their websites are full of information which is both generic and national. The RNIB does benefit checks and both societies do phone counselling. All services are now free for those two charities.

- There are a number of local and national charities that have grant schemes for people with sight loss. Find out more about grants from other organisations. http://www.rnib.org.uk/information-everyday-living-benefits-and-concessions-grants/grants-other-organisations
- The RNIB offers grants of up to £500 for certain small items of technology to people who are registered as blind or partially sighted, on a means-tested benefit and who have been unable to get statutory funding. Read about grants from RNIB and how you can apply for a grant for yourself or your VIP (http://www.rnib.org.uk/information-everyday-living-benefits-and-concessions-grants/grants-rnib).
- If your VIP is interested in music equipment, lessons, study or activities, take a look at the RNIB's information about music awards and funding. http://www.rnib.org.uk/information-everyday-living-home-and-leisure-music/music-awards-and-funding

While on these sites for generic information, you can also burrow down to the local level to see what is available where you live.

I will mention again a particularly good source of help via the RNIB/Action for Blind, namely, the courses called 'Finding your Feet.' See Chapter 8 to remind yourself of the details.

You will soon begin to realise that local provision is variable. There is no consistency in what is provided by either councils or charities. It is difficult to give good advice, therefore, apart from getting out and investigating. The variety of what's on offer is down to the motivation, skill level and experience of the local organisers and volunteers. They may be highly professional and knowledgeable, or they may be completely misguided and hopeless.

Please don't be put off by bad experiences with one organisation. You may get what you need at the next. The provision of help for those with MD is a

Cinderella service. If the council provision is poor, then often this will spark the voluntary sector to 'fill in the gaps', or vice versa.

You will begin to realise that a lot of effort for the blind and partially sighted is expended to help those who may need employment, i.e. younger people of working age or young children. Frustratingly, these groups are a small percentage of those with visual loss, but a lot more money is expended on them. MD is the sad orphan, in terms of resources directed to help its sufferers. It is not a sexy disease, although in percentage terms it's the largest cause of vision loss in the UK.

When looking for help, do use the local library, as well as Google. It is a good starting point. Small local groups are not always good at providing an internet presence, so the library can be good to get an overview of local provision. Ask at the desk. They are likely to have lists of local organisations and events that may be happening.

Finally, check noticeboards in post offices, shops, supermarkets, or in church halls or village and community halls – anywhere people gather together. These noticeboards will suggest which groups are alive and kicking in your area. Ask, too, at your local GP surgery.

You need to keep your eyes and ears open for any information about local help. It may masquerade under many banners. Also look out for carers' organisations for you to attend. These can be invaluable for getting advice and information about what is going on in your area. There is bound to be stuff happening wherever you live, but it can feel a bit subterranean. You need to resemble a truffle hound.

In Touch on BBC Radio 4 is a regular weekly programme for the blind and partially sighted. It has run for many years, but because of its long history it doesn't tend to discuss basic problems. It is more of an up-to-the-minute magazine format, with advice, news, etc. It may seem a bit 'pick and mix' if you only listen once, but if you listen in the longer term you will get lots of really useful information. There is an accompanying website with follow-up information, and BBC iPlayer has the entire back catalogue, amounting to several hundred programmes.

A final source of information is the Sightline Directory (sightline.org.uk), which acts as a portal to many websites and organisations.

Look out for:

- Local travel schemes
- Buddy schemes
- Volunteering schemes (RNIB)
- Age UK groups for help with shopping
- Access technology to use kit easily
- Talking magazines (http://www.tnauk.org.uk)
- Everyday Solutions magazine catalogue has a lot of useful stuff

Read up about all the available assistance at home before venturing into the territory of Social Services. When with professionals, keep asking questions. What is available? From whom and where? How can you get what, and when?

KEY POINTS

- You have to be fairly assertive in your approach to organisations. It is easy to be rebuffed, particularly by Social Services, when your VIP may well be entitled to something. This is where you may need to be assertive in getting him what should be his by right.

- You have to be persistent. Like a terrier at a bone, don't let go, until you have at least got something.

- Sightline directory (sightline.org.uk) acts as a portal to many websites and organisations.

- For up to date information on benefits and support go to the RNIB website: https://www.rnib.org.uk/benefits-and-support

- Listen to Radio 4's In Touch for the latest information, tips and advice

- Keep your eyes and ears open for local charities/services.

Help is out there – trust me – but you may need to be curious, assertive and persistent to discover it.

PART THREE

Every day is a journey, and
the journey itself is home

– Matsuo Basho

A place for everything and
everything in its place

– Mrs Beeton, The Book of Household Management

Please put everything back in exactly the same place you found it.

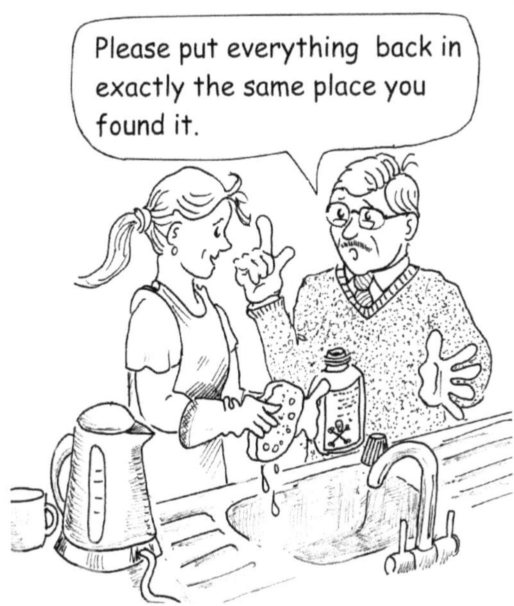

CHAPTER 13

Around The Home

Home is where the VIP will spend most of her time and where she will want to 'do' things. Homes are our most personal spaces and are where our habits are most deeply entrenched.

Therefore, the VIP's home is likely to be the place that poses the most difficult problems.

Life at home should be easy, safe and enjoyable – but a change in vision can wreak havoc on a place that ought to be a refuge.

There is a conflict for the VIP when it comes to her home. She wants to continue with her life as it has always been. The alternative is to change behaviour patterns and try something new, but any changes in behaviour are difficult, as we've seen, because the VIP's brain is already fried, simply from coping with her loss of vision.

When we are under stress, most of us retreat into our shells and seek comfort. VIPs are no different.

Trying to change someone's patterns of behaviour is an area fraught with potential pitfalls. **You can't just dive in and start changing things.** Be warned: home is where the toddler VIP can be at her grumpiest.

There is an old joke about a crowd of poker players in a smoke-filled room. Someone walks in and says, 'This place is full of smoke, you need to open a window,' to which one of the players replies, 'How do you know? You only just walked in here.'

Life with a VIP can be a bit like that. You, the coach, can see blatant problems that the VIP is unaware of. This is where a simple chat comes in. What's bugging her? What is difficult, dangerous or just annoying?

One of the problems you may encounter is that the VIP will have adapted to a certain extent. She will have found her own ways to do things, just about. She is likely to be embarrassed about not being able to do 'simple' things. You may find that she can't imagine there is any other way of doing something that she has done in the same way for 75 years.

Listen to what your VIP wants. Make a list of things she is struggling with, then tackle them one by one. Don't go for something difficult to start with. Go for the quick wins. Small changes, completed straightforwardly, will make life easier.

Once one change is absorbed, move on to the next. Create the 'virtuous circle'. Free up some of her overworked brain cells. She will be able to take on more challenges as life gets easier.

As time goes on, you may deal with the more deep-seated problems. These will be more time-consuming, expensive, or complex to handle. They may need more thought and planning. Grab the low-hanging fruit first.

This is a difficult chapter to write, as everyone has different problems and, of course, different homes. It is impossible to cover all the potential pitfalls of life with vision loss, but there are common problems that seem to recur with many VIPs, so these are my general suggestions.

My number one suggestion applies to all VIPs, and it is this: **arrange a home visit from a ROVI / Occupational Therapist** (their full title is Rehabilitation Officer for People with a Vision Impairment). ROVIs are a great bunch of people. The main problem is finding one. They are usually employed by Social Services departments or charities for blind and partially sighted people. They may also work in hospitals, day care and residential services.

Try your local Social Services department first, or go to your local council's website. They will have dedicated workers for blind and partially sighted people. These workers may or may not be ROVIs.

If Social Services can't help, try any local visual impaired charities. They may employ ROVIs or know who does. If you attend an Action for Blind course, they should know of ROVIs in the area.

What you really want is a ROVI who will come to the home. A home visit is invaluable in providing information and suggestions. The ROVI will have a lot of practical suggestions and tips.

She will have a look around the home for areas that could be improved, or where additional equipment would help. She will be concerned with safety in the home, initially, and then with how well the room works, concentrating on the bathroom and kitchen. The ROVI can help with existing equipment, making it simpler to use, or she may suggest new equipment.

She will also make assessments, if she works for Social Services. This may help you get further help for your VIP. The ROVI can put you in touch with further organisations or with departments who can offer more help.

She will have a lot of experience in assessing homes. She can draw up a list of improvements and possible modifications; things that would take a long time to occur to the average layman.

The other advantage of a ROVI is she will be seen as an expert. Her advice (which may be exactly the same as yours) will be believed and acted on by the VIP. This will feel slightly galling if you have been suggesting something for months, something that is now suddenly seized on as a good idea by the VIP. ROVIs can be a useful means of moving people on from old habits.

Make sure you are there when the ROVI turns up to make the most of her expertise (ROVIs do tend to be female). Two people asking questions will make the visit more useful, and together you're more likely to remember the information after she has left.

The ROVI is likely to suggest ideas for improvement in the following categories:

- Safety around the home
- Organisational discipline
- De-cluttering
- Lighting
- Cooking/eating
- Communication
- Television
- Paperwork

A visit from the ROVI can be a great way to kickstart your VIP in getting motivated for action.

1. Safety

Safety in the home is extremely important and should be looked at as soon as possible. It is bad enough having poor vision; you don't want to add an avoidable accident in the home to your VIP's problems.

The home needs to be risk-assessed, which is jargon for having a walk around and looking critically for potential hazards.

While you are assessing safety, think about the home functionally. Is it easy to work in? The two most important rooms are the bathroom and the kitchen; we cannot function without them. These rooms need to be easy to work in, free of clutter, and with space to put things in an orderly way.

- Electrical appliances and fixtures need to be safe. No loose wiring or badly wired plugs, and minimal extension leads, which should be out of the way when walking.
- The floor should be free of trip hazards. No rugs that flip over or carpets with edges that ruck up. The pet basket and feed saucers should be kept in clearly defined areas, not on a walking route.
- Any stairs need to be clutter-free, and non-slip with handrails. It is easier to lose balance with poor sight.
- If there are glass doors, you may need to replace them or get them marked. Otherwise it is easy to walk into them without realising they are there.

The obvious problem that arises here is the shower room. Any glass door around the shower may need to have a coloured stripe fitted across it at eye level. This may apply in other parts of a home, too, for instance, the conservatory or garden doors. Fitting visibility stripes can be done to fit in with the decor, but the primary function is visibility. We have all seen those pratfall clips of people walking into glass doors on the TV – and those are people with good vision.

I hate to say it, but try the exercise with the Vaseline glasses and then go around the VIP's home and do a few routine tasks. This will show up potential hazards quickly. While you are about it, try and prepare some food wearing the glasses, as a way of identifying problem areas in the kitchen.

2. Organisational discipline

The simplest and most important thing to do to make life easier is free, but it is one of the most difficult to implement. Being organised is always a good habit; in the fight against MD, it becomes crucial. This covers everything from where you keep your scissors to legal issues like making a will.

This is a case of do as I say, not as I do. I am naturally untidy and disorganised. A friend of mine once described my organisational skills as 'the deep litter system of management'. With me, everything is there should you need it, but you have to burrow through a ton of stuff to track it down.

It is therefore ironic that I am urging you to do something I don't do myself. If I had a diagnosis of MD, I would have to change my habits radically, and it would hurt.

I am in the habit of casually using articles and then discarding them wherever I happen to be. Correspondence I put down in the general direction of my desk.

With MD, if you put something down in a random place it will disappear. The VIP will spend many, many hours fruitlessly searching for stuff that is under her nose. The frustration in such situations can be unbearable, knowing something is within reach but being unable to locate it.

Mrs Beeton is right: everything should have a place. You need to be tyrannical in your insistence on this. Instil discipline in your VIP about always putting an object in its designated place. Then, when she goes back to that place, she will find what she wants. (This may lead to tense negotiations about which drawer the Sellotape should live in and a debate about why you keep the dog biscuits in a particular cupboard.)

However, beware: if you discussed this with me I would see the logic, agree wholeheartedly and listen to the suggestions. Two days later I would still be putting the Sellotape back on the shelf in the wrong room.

What makes this even more difficult is that you must get ***everybody else*** in the home to exercise this iron discipline. If you as a coach use something, you, too, must replace it in its permanent place. In the long run, organisational discipline will make life much easier for everyone. Without it, stress levels in the home will reach crisis point quickly and often.

Visitors can be disastrous to a household in this respect. They may tidy up and put stuff away in an effort to be helpful. Where they put something will be logical to them, but the VIP may find she's lost it for weeks before it turns up. You need to explain this to everyone who enters the home. It is not obsessive tidiness; it is a system to stop the VIP going nuts, and everyone has to comply.

Dump spots

On the organisation of personal belongings – keys, purse, wallet, the stuff we need daily – I would recommend having three 'dump' areas where they are left, one by the front door, one in the bedroom, and maybe one in the kitchen.

When your VIP comes home tired, she must simply drop stuff off into those spots. Then, when she needs to find it again, it should be in one of the drop-off zones, rather than just casually left somewhere that seemed convenient at the time.

Iron discipline with this kind of household organisation won't be easy, but if implemented it will reduce a lot of unnecessary stress and wasted time.

3. De-cluttering

This is the identical twin of organisational discipline.

It is something most of us agree with in principle, but never quite get around to doing. Some people successfully delay this until after they reach death's door.

I would not suggest putting a de-clutter at the top of a to-do list for the recently visually impaired. It may be far too traumatic in the early days, but some way down the line it would be really helpful.

Put simply: the less stuff there is cluttering up the home, the easier it is to find what you want. We all have stuff that seems gradually to adhere to us, the man- or woman-drawer with 'useful' stuff that has been there for years.

The ideal situation is one in which you can go to the drawer and immediately put your hand on what you want. You don't want to rummage around for ten minutes amongst a load of rubbish, half of which has no real use anyway.

To achieve this, reduce the number of things that are there. It's that simple.

We all know the drill for de-cluttering. Pick a drawer, and then:

- Empty the drawer.
- Put back only those things that are used.
- Everything else goes to the dump or a charity shop.

You should then have a manageable number of things in the drawer. Job done.

Repeat for all drawers, cupboards, shelves throughout the house. You may allow yourself the odd sentimental item.

Start a de-clutter with clothing

Rather than threaten the VIP with, 'I am going to throw away all this rubbish you've collected,' a subtler way to introduce this topic is to suggest you go through her clothes. Don't use the word 'de-cluttering.' Instead, try, 'How about sorting your clothes so you can find things more easily?' Or, 'We could sort out matching outfits?' Or, 'Let's separate your winter clothes from your summer ones.' Any excuse will do.

Particularly for women, selecting clothes from a wardrobe can be difficult with poor vision. Arranging dresses, skirts or suits in some form of order so that your VIP can find matching outfits is helpful.

This is a way of de-cluttering by the back door. While sorting through clothes, you can helpfully check each item is OK. If things are damaged or worn out, get rid of them. The VIP may be unaware of how each piece has deteriorated over time. She won't see the worn cuffs or collars. As for stuff that doesn't fit any longer, or is out of fashion, or that needs repairs, or that doesn't suit her? Pieces that haven't been worn for a couple of years? Get rid of it all.

We have all seen old people looking dishevelled and tatty, but often it is not because they don't care. It is because they don't know what they look like.

Having filtered out all the old, damaged, not-relevant stuff, make sure what's left is organised within its drawers, on shelves, racks etc. Create a system for selecting outfits that will leave your VIP with fewer items to rummage through. This sounds easy, but can take a lot of time.

If in doubt buy a book about de-cluttering – but don't let it add to the original clutter!

De-cluttering clothes makes getting dressed much easier for your VIP. It helps her to find clothes quickly and efficiently. It also takes away those doubts about her personal presentation when in public.

When you have 'done' her clothing, you can move on to other areas. For women, a similar exercise may be useful for jewellery. Select items that can easily be used with simple clasps or fittings. Keep these separate. More difficult-to-use pieces may be put away for special occasions when help is at hand.

Your second target for de-cluttering is the kitchen.

Drawers of implements and odds and ends tend to build up in our kitchens. Again, you need to be ruthless. It is unlikely your VIP will be cooking gourmet dinner parties for ten. Get the basics sorted out: kitchen knives, openers, spatulas, stuff you would need in a basic student/camping kitchen. The other, more esoteric stuff (asparagus steamers, butter curling tongs) relegate to a box that your VIP can rummage through if she really has to.

Then clear out the cupboards. Eliminate any excess crockery, leaving just the basics easily to hand.

Finally, sort out the food cupboards. Clear out old jars of coffee and spices or herbs with sell-by dates from three years ago.

You get the idea. *Simplify.* You don't want your VIP faffing around for ten minutes just working out which can of soup she wants.

This de-clutter could take months in practice, but if you gradually work from room to room or pile to pile, appropriately and with consideration, it will be time well spent.

Finally, a slightly underhand but effective tip. Many years ago, I had a friend whose wife was a compulsive hoarder. When he wanted to get rid of stuff he would clear out his wife's unwanted clutter and put it in the dustbin.

The trick, though, was to put it in his neighbour's dustbin. If he put it in his own, his wife would just remove it and carry it back into the house. Please use your discretion with this practice though; you want to rid the house of real clutter and rubbish, not cherished possessions.

4. Lighting

With lighting, the rules for an easy-to-use room are simple:

- Good lighting
- Good contrast

Good lighting

Wherever your VIP undertakes tasks, there should be good lighting. This can be a simple desk-type lamp; a fixture, preferably, but floor-standing or on a worktop will also do. This applies in the bedroom, kitchen, bathroom – everywhere needs to be flooded with light.

I have no strong feelings about different types of lighting. Individual lights should be bright and easily directed, and if a light is going to be near the VIP it should not be hot to the touch. LED lights provide all of the above and are cheap to run. An individual LED lamp won't give full room lighting, but for specific tasks they are usually best.

There are hundreds of types of lamps and light bulbs available, but the simple rule of thumb is the stronger the light the better, both physically and in the amount of light given out.

You may see adverts for daylight bulbs in Saturday supplements and other publications. You can spend a fortune on some of these lamps and daylight bulbs. I would recommend you try before you buy. I am not convinced of their superiority but if it works for your VIP that is all that matters.

In a reading area, the double 'mother-and-child' type lamps are very good, with the 'mother' lighting the room generally, while the 'child' shines on the reading matter. In a kitchen environment or bedroom, a simple desk or freestanding LED lamp works well. Bathrooms must have some form of fitted lamp for safety reasons.

Grab your Vaseline glasses and wander around the home looking at dials and knobs and packets in various places. Then try looking at each item with more light. You will quickly realise the difference you can make.

- If something can't be lit easily, for instance, in a bathroom, consider an LED torch. Small rechargeable lithium torches are very powerful, and some can be carried on a key ring.
- Wherever there is a problem with viewing detail, leave a torch in place for your VIP.

Good contrast

For VIPs, the loss of visual detail effectively camouflages objects against their backgrounds.

The surface light falls on is therefore important to make their life easier. Worktops and flat surfaces are best in simple, plain colours. White with no patterns works best for seeing things clearly.

Wooden or patterned effects are difficult for VIPs. What you are looking for is the maximum contrast between the surface and any objects. A quick solution is to cover surfaces with a plain white cloth to make it easier to see.

The kitchen is a place where your VIP will want to reach for and use something quickly, without thinking about it. Often kitchens are colour-coordinated, which looks lovely; however, those matching sets of jars containing tea, coffee, sugar, salt, flour etc, are a minefield. If your VIP wants to keep them, stick large, coloured labels on them.

I recommend that you replace things that are difficult to see. Clear drinking glasses, for instance, are difficult to pick up if you can't see them. Replace them with a coloured version, or change the material. Plastic is ideal as it bounces (although people often don't like the feel of plastic for drinking).

6. Cooking

This is probably the area where you can help most as a coach. We all have to eat something, but poor vision creates a multitude of intersecting problems when it comes to preparing and eating food.

Although this is an important area, it is difficult to give specific advice as people's diets are so varied. So much depends on what your VIP has been used to cooking and eating. Food preparation methods differ with every household, ranging from the gourmet cook to the takeaway junkie.

It can be all too easy for a lone individual to gently starve herself when poor vision comes into play. Some VIPs find they can't be bothered to prepare food at all. It is simply too much effort, particularly if they live alone. Or they may exist on what they can zap in the microwave, finding anything else too difficult. Mull over what your VIP's diet is like and whether it is the act of cooking that is a problem for her, perhaps because her late partner used to do it all, or perhaps because she now can't cope with the equipment or skills required to prepare a meal.

Shopping is covered in a separate chapter, so for now we will assume your VIP has whatever is needed in her store cupboards.

Let's break down food preparation to its basics. Your VIP must:

- Select the ingredients for a meal
- Prepare these ingredients for cooking
- Cook in some way (or not, if served cold)
- Serve up for eating

This may seem simplistic but let's work through this process for a simple snack – say, beans on toast – as though we were a VIP.

First we select the ingredients: a tin of beans, bread and butter.

Baked beans. But which tin is the baked beans? Rummaging around in the cupboard for a tin that is not soup, fruit or some other vegetable can take time. Does your VIP have a system for distinguishing between six different red cans of soup, all with different flavours?

Bread: ready-sliced, probably. But has it gone off? Are there mouldy bits on it?

Butter: select from fridge. But which is the right carton? The right package?

Having found our ingredients, let's prepare them.

Opening the tin of beans is not so easy with poor vision, especially if a tin-opener is involved. The cans with a quick-release top are better, but your VIP will still need to be cautious with the edges.

Now we cook the meal.

Let's prepare the beans on the hob. Are the temperature dials easy to use? How long should we cook the beans for? It's hard to tell when you can't see.

Meanwhile, we toast the bread. Smell is helpful here. You know by smell when you have burnt the toast. A fool-proof toaster is a helpful addition to your VIP's kitchen.

Now we butter the toast. Spreadable butter is easier than traditional solid butter from the fridge, but try buttering toast with the Vaseline glasses on; it really is difficult to judge how much butter you are using and how effectively you have spread it.

See how a simple snack is suddenly much more complicated than normal? Now imagine how those problems would multiply if we had been cooking a full meal from scratch.

A lot of people do carry on cooking from basic ingredients with poor vision. But you can understand why there is a tendency to go straight to the microwave meal. The majority of VIPs use microwavable or ready meals. Sadly, the old meals on wheels delivery service has been killed off by the microwave in most of the country.

But by using the techniques of brainstorming and playing to concentrate on the process of cooking, rather than the results, you can make real progress in the kitchen with your VIP. You can help her regain enough confidence to tackle jobs in the kitchen again.

Start a conversation with her about what she wants to eat, and perhaps what she misses eating. Then brainstorm for solutions and have fun in the kitchen trying out new ideas. One lady I know switched to red-skinned potatoes so she'd know whether she had peeled them properly. Simple yet effective solutions like this one can make a big difference.

I sometimes joke that Americans are better than the British at cooking. This can irritate people slightly, but there is a reason for the statement.

A British recipe uses weight measurements. An American version uses volumes. So instead of 8oz of flour, 4oz of sugar and half a pint of milk, the American recipe would call for 2 cups of flour, 1 cup of sugar and a mug of milk.

If you cook in the British way, you have to use scales. With American recipes, you fill up containers. To transition to the US method, you would weigh out 4 ounces of flour, but then find a mug or small bowl that the 4 ounces fills to the brim. From then on, that recipe would call for 'the mug with the flowers on' (for instance) to supply your 4 ounces. You can repeat this so that your VIP has a series of containers that she knows will always give her the required amounts.

You can also buy American cup-style measuring containers in kitchen shops or online. This means converting favourite recipes to volumes, rather than the traditional weight measurements. This switch requires some effort. If you convert old recipes one by one, over time it will make cooking easier and the cakes will taste just the same.

It is also a good idea to look at the variety of your VIP's diet. Nobody wants to eat pot noodles every day of their lives.

Above all, time spent brainstorming recipes in the kitchen will help your VIP regain her confidence in the kitchen. She can learn new ways of getting the results she wants. If you are lucky there may even be cooking courses for the visually impaired locally (the provision of this type of course is rare, unfortunately).

Concerns about safety and food may mean you are contemplating a kitchen refit. A refit is a great way of making life easier and simpler for your VIP, if it is carefully thought through. Please don't employ a kitchen fitter simply to make things look nice. You need someone who is going to take time to think about what it would be like to operate with poor vision. Try him or her with the Vaseline glasses!

A kitchen fitter could suggest all sorts of equipment that may be helpful for your VIP. One such example is an induction hob. These heat by magnetic induction. The hob only stays hot if there is a metal pot on it. Induction hobs are super-efficient and easy to clean. They act almost like a gas hob, but the main advantage is safety. The VIP is much less likely to burn herself.

You may also want to consider installing controls that don't require you to reach over the hob. Someone with poor vision may need to lean in close to check the settings – not a good idea with a traditional cooker.

Go to https://www.cobolt.co.uk/ for more about a talking induction hob for VIPs. Brilliant.

Cooking and kitchen safety is one area where the ROVI will be able to give invaluable advice. She understands the importance of making sure your VIP has a good balanced diet for her overall health. She might have ideas and recommendations should you opt for a kitchen refit.

7. Communications

It is vital to make sure your VIP can communicate with the outside world. The phone is her lifeline. While most people use mobiles these days, which are great when your vision is good, the size of the average mobile phone makes it a difficult option for VIPs. The good, old-fashioned landline is still best at home, preferably with large buttons – the bigger the better.

Even if your VIP lives with someone who has good vision, the landline is a vital piece of equipment you should aim to change. After all, your VIP may need to make an emergency call for her partner sometime.

You should also aim to get the phone numbers she uses regularly formatted in large print. This list can then be kept near the phone. It is worth doing this even if the numbers are already pre-programmed into the phone.

8. Television

While we are on the subject of your VIP's house, let's discuss the TV. If you were deaf you would turn up the sound on your set and nobody would be surprised, but few people bother to turn up the 'vision' on their TV.

If you want to see a TV more easily, adjust the set. On the remote control in the centre is a 'menu' button that is rarely used. If you press this button it should bring up three controls:

- Colour
- Brightness
- Contrast

These three will let you adjust the picture. You will need the VIP's input on this. Adjust the slider controls for these three menu options. You may think the picture looks terrible, but the VIP can tell you when she's able to see it better. It takes a bit of fiddling around to get the best result, but it's worth the effort.

Also on the subject of the TV, would a bigger, better-quality set be a good investment? Take a trip to a shop that sells TVs, just to look at some options. It costs nothing, and the VIP may be surprised how well she can see with some of the new screens available. A small diversion on your next shopping trip is worth the waste of a few minutes.

The simplest way to improve the picture on TV, however, is to move the VIP's chair nearer to the TV or the TV nearer to her chair. If you halve the distance between them it doubles the size of the image. Twice as much TV for no cost at all!

9. Paperwork and post

There is a constant blizzard of mail to people's homes nowadays. Most of it is junk mail, but even this has to be dealt with. When I pick up my post I recognise the junk from the real stuff and bin the junk immediately.

Sometimes, though, I'm unsure about certain envelopes. I have to open them to check whether they're junk or not. If you can't see, this quick sorting system becomes more difficult. Each piece of mail has to be opened and assessed before binning.

It may be that your VIP needs someone else to open and deal with her mail. Personal, intimate correspondence and financial information can be sensitive topics, however; whoever takes on this task must be chosen by the VIP, and it needs to be someone she trusts. There can be no discussion on this. The VIP's decision is final as to who reads her most intimate correspondence.

Contact utility companies

Your VIP can maintain control of her finances for longer if you arrange for utilities and regular bills to be sent in large-print format. Organisations don't care whether bills are sent out in normal print or large print; once they hit the computer button it will churn out correspondence as instructed, at no inconvenience to the company.

One happy side effect of requesting large print bills is that it becomes easier to sort out junk mail, as junk envelopes won't be addressed in large print.

Bills and invoices can also be sent online. Most utilities, credit card companies, etc, are happy to send emails instead of paper bills. Just ask them. If your VIP doesn't do so already, consider switching her payments to direct debit – all in the cause of making life easier.

Joe's story

Bryan was a good friend of Joe's. They lived in the same village. Since Bryan's retirement, he'd taken care to look out for the old man, who had been on his own following his wife's death. Bryan knew Joe was struggling. Joe complained bitterly about not being able to read his books about tanks. He had been in the tank corps as a young man.

Joe was becoming a bit of a recluse. He would sit around for hours and was no longer going out. The garden was becoming overgrown, whereas previously Joe had spent most of the day pottering about on his vegetable plot. The garden had provided most of the couple's fruit and veg when Joe's wife was still alive.

Joe had taken his wife's death badly, and the loss of his sight was the final straw as far as he was concerned. Bryan had been a social worker before his retirement, so he knew how to judge when someone was struggling, but he knew nothing about visual loss.

The two men came to see me and we discussed the situation. They decided to put in place some changes slowly over the next three months, at which point we would review Joe's case.

The first change Bryan implemented was quick and easy. He shifted Joe's chair five feet forward towards the TV. This doesn't sound much, but the distance was half what it had been before, and it instantly made the television much easier to see. The screen was effectively twice as big. The second thing Bryan did was to introduce Joe to the Yesterday channel, which shows a lot of war-related programmes.

Over the next few weeks, Bryan gradually introduced more changes. The RNIB online shop provided a large button telephone for £20. Joe had a cordless one before, but he kept losing it. He went back to a corded phone so he'd know where it was all the time. The large buttons were easier for him to use, not because the numbers were bigger, but because he could feel his way around the key pad with his fingers. Bryan programmed in his own number, the doctor's and those of Joe's children who lived away. The two men had a session playing around with it one morning, and then Bryan got Joe to phone him regularly to make sure he had mastered the keypad.

They took a trip to the bank and asked for all Joe's bank statements to be sent out in large print in future. Joe listened politely to the bank clerk explaining internet banking and decided not to take up her kind offer. He was less polite to Bryan when they got outside. 'Bloody internet this and internet that, what do I want that for?'

As Joe's bills came in from the utility companies and the council, they gradually converted them to big print. This involved more military language from Joe as he wrestled with his new phone and the bureaucracy involved. Being ex-military, he was not going to go down without fighting back.

I had given Joe a couple of magnifying glasses when I saw him and he began using these around the house. He could read the television times in the newspaper and the cooking directions on packets of food. He kept the larger one with a light in it by his chair. The little one he kept in his pocket to whip out whenever he needed it.

He also ordered a subscription to the 'big print newspaper' from the RNIB. This was a success. Joe didn't like the newspaper, but he loved the television and radio supplement in large print. He could read this without the use of a magnifier.

KEY POINTS

- Find a ROVI locally and arrange a home visit
- Check for any safety hazards around the home
- Work gradually on the tasks that are really causing problems for your VIP
- Food is one area where you can experiment with brainstorming and play exercises. Have some fun in the kitchen with the VIP

I'm sorry if this chapter has been rather preachy, but changing habits is difficult and requires time and a lot of patience. Everybody in the household will be affected. If you need to reorganise, others are going to notice and you may well experience some resistance.

It's important that other members of the household understand what you are doing and why. It's a difficult balance, but you do have to accommodate the needs of other family members – it is their home as well.

Technology is a gift of God. After the gift of life it is perhaps the greatest of God's gifts. It is the mother of civilisations, of arts and of sciences

– Freeman Dyson

Wow !
With the font enlarged
I can read my e-mails.

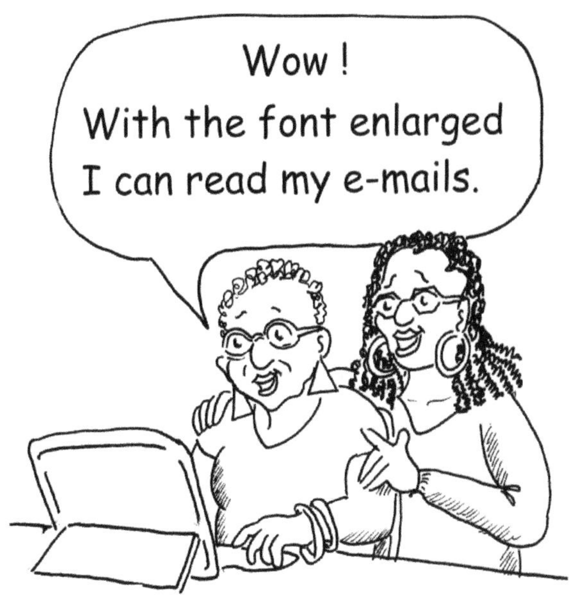

CHAPTER 14

Technology

There are major potential benefits for VIPs if you are able to find the right piece of equipment. What I mean by technology is really any object that can be used to do a job. This may be a piece of software, an app, or a device to detect whether you have filled a cup enough.

The digital age has transformed our lives. Most of us have a love/hate relationship with technology. We love sending emails, Skype, buying tickets and goods online, playing games, watching television.

We hate it when the printer won't work. We hate it when unknown people try to befriend us on Facebook, or when we get locked into a horrendous loop whilst trying to buy stuff on the internet.

Ideally, technology needs to give maximum help with minimum frustration.

People vary enormously in their enthusiasm for technology, whatever their age. Their ability to cope with it depends on their motivation. If they can be shown a good enough reason to use something, most people are willing to learn how it works.

VIPs tend to be wary of technology, and with good reason. If an item is going to be used by someone with poor vision it needs to be bombproof, both in its ease of use and its reliability. If you struggle to cope with an item when you have good vision, it will likely be useless for those with MD.

This chapter therefore comes with a health warning: technology has downsides as well as upsides. Remember the acronym KISS (keep it simple, stupid).

For our purposes there are two types of technology – the normal stuff used by everyone and the stuff designed specifically for visually impaired people.

Let's deal with the normal stuff that your VIP probably owns already.

Every home has an assortment of electric appliances and equipment. The majority will have been there a while and the VIP will be used to using them.

Some items may have become more difficult to use since your VIP's vision changed, and others will need replacing due to obsolescence or because they've broken down. A cull is probably a good idea. You may have started on this already, if you did a de-clutter earlier.

Ask yourself, can the VIP still use this piece of equipment with poor vision? He may have had his microwave for ten years, but have stopped using it because he can no longer see the controls.

Set up a 'play time' with any equipment your VIP is struggling with or not using. He can practise using it by feeling his way around the controls. With the microwave, 'waste' a microwave meal, or just boil some water for tea. (Be careful, though; water can explode in a microwave if over-heated; in itself a good reason to practise).

Technology is one area where ROVIs are invaluable. They know how to make equipment more user-friendly, how to adapt things, or what changes might be necessary.

If equipment needs replacing, I am a great fan of cheap appliances. For the VIP, the cheapest may be best. The reason is not cost, but because cheap devices normally have fewer programs and buttons.

Buy the item with the least number of buttons. The ultimate appliance is a one-button job, off or on. The more buttons, the more complicated it is for the VIP. Our aim with any new technology is to reduce confusion.

Don't be seduced by sophistication; it won't help, and the appliance will most likely be side-lined. Your VIP may come up with excuses as to why it is not used, when in reality it is too complicated. Getting a new piece of kit is a learning curve for anybody; for those with poor sight it is a series of hairpin bends up a mountain.

One of the unintended consequences of the digital revolution is that it has a downside for VIPs. Buttons and dials are becoming increasingly obsolete. Touch screen controls are now becoming ubiquitous, but these are difficult to operate if you can't see what to touch.

Visit www.abilitynet.org.uk for lots of great information about different technologies and equipment. When buying, go online for up-to-date information about suppliers, prices, etc. This chapter cannot be comprehensive in that respect, because there is always something new coming out.

However, there are basics that don't change much over time and they can be found easily. Your first port of call should be the RNIB online shop (http://shop.rnib.org.uk/), which supplies items from telephones to white sticks. The shop is a useful starting point. A visit can help stimulate your thoughts and can lead to a discussion as to what could help your VIP.

You might then wish to try more specialised firms for specific items. There are a lot of potentially helpful devices. Some are easy to use, while others need more time and skill.

Start with the easy stuff first. The following equipment is likely to be useful to most VIPs and all items are easy to use immediately.

- Talking watches/clocks
- Specialist lights
- Large buttoned telephones
- Talking bathroom scales
- Remote controls for TV and radio

Pick an easy win. A good start is a talking watch or a large button phone. Most people are pleased to have a basic task made easier.

Most of the equipment in the list works either by making the controls bigger to handle or by making them audible.

Making things bigger has two effects. First, obviously, your VIP can see them more easily. The second effect is less obvious. It has to do with muscle memory.

We drive a car using muscle memory. We know how it feels to change from second to third gear without thinking about it. If the actions are slightly more pronounced (i.e. because we're using a bigger piece of equipment), they tend to be more easily remembered. We're back to the subject of 'fast thinking.' We want to get your VIP using his devices with hardly any conscious thought at all.

The operation of the device is critical. It should be simple and intuitive in use. If it's not, choose something else. Remember your VIP's limited brain energy. He is likely exhausted from just getting through the day. Try operating any new equipment yourself with your eyes closed before buying.

This second, more specialised list of equipment contains items that are more difficult to master, though in the longer term though they make life more enjoyable.

- DAB radio
- Audiobook readers
- Voice recorders
- Labelling devices
- Talking tape measures

DAB radios

A DAB radio can be a very welcome addition to the home, if your VIP doesn't already have one. DAB gives the advantage of a much wider range of stations to listen to. Instead of being stuck on one station, your VIP can switch easily between several stations of a similar type. Take some time to investigate stations that might appeal to your VIP's usual listening habits. The selection of stations is precise with DAB. There's no fiddling around to tune the radio, and similar stations are often grouped together when you turn the dial. Radio is a good friend to the partially sighted.

You probably don't need to buy a new radio, as most TVs now stream radio through the set. But this is often overlooked by people who aren't used to it and who think of the TV as just the 'telly'.

Audiobook readers

Audiobook readers come in a wide variety of styles. Originally these were simple tape recorders, but they have moved on through all sorts of formats, and the latest incarnations use USB sticks. This is great for the supplier – It makes it easier to supply and copy material, and they are user-friendly. The advantage of USB sticks is that they can be easily copied.

These are available through the RNIB at a cost of about £25. You simply plug in the USB stick to the dedicated player. But first check what your local library supplies by way of talking books, CDs or USB?

Talking magazines and newspapers (national as well as local) are also available, as are audio books. If you go online you can find the where, who and how to contact for talking newspapers.

Listening to an audiobook – whether it is a novel or a newspaper – sounds easy, but your VIP may have to learn how to use one to get the most out of it. When we read a good book we often say we 'get lost in it'. That is because the story grips us. We get caught up, to the extent that the real world almost ceases to exist.

With an audiobook, it isn't so easy to get into that wonderful imaginative state. The audiobook bowls along at the pace of the actor reading it, and you have to keep up with him. Sometimes he leaves you behind. An audiobook doesn't give you the opportunity to pause for breath from reading, or to contemplate what you have just heard and puzzle out what is going on. With an audiobook murder mystery, for instance, it's easy to miss the clues that would help solve the murder.

Your VIP will have to train himself to listen actively (as opposed to the casual listening which we tend to use when the radio is playing away in the background). He may find he needs to stop, pause, and restart the audio regularly, particularly if he is listening to a factual book.

Due to the limited concentration span of the VIP, though, it's quite likely he will doze off after listening to a story or article for just a few minutes, and then come to, having no idea of where he needs to get back to in the recording. If this happens regularly, he is likely to give up on audiobooks. As coach, you can help him to understand that he may need to limit his listening time. He will also need to learn to use the controls on the recording equipment properly so that he can find his way back into the story.

Having mentioned talking newspapers, it is worth mentioning here one of my favourite publications, the large print newspaper. This is a national newspaper in, as you may have guessed, LARGE PRINT. The reason I particularly like it is because of its great weekly TV and radio supplement. The large print newspaper is available through the RNIB. Just look on their website for it. It is delivered by post weekly for a small cost.

Voice recorders

The voice recorder is not an obvious choice when you have good vision. But imagine your weekly food shop. First, you need to know what you are going to buy. Before I go shopping I will go into the kitchen and look in the cupboards to see what we need. I then write a shopping list – not necessarily an option for your VIP.

The voice recorder is a great tool for reminders and lists for your VIP. He can carry it around with him and record messages for himself ('*a can of cat food, some toilet rolls and toothpaste*'). He can also record appointments ('*Dentist check-up, Tuesday the 8th*'; '*Meet Jenny in Starbucks 11.00am Saturday*'). The voice recorder is an audible notebook. It is a very useful device, but it is a different way of working from a bit of paper and may take some getting used to.

The RNIB does a great little voice recorder which costs about £199. It fits in the pocket and is easy to use.

The labelling device RNIB PenFriend 2 is a voice recorder labeller and an interesting device. A sighted person would never consider it, but for a VIP it can be very helpful.

Again, think about going shopping and the business of deciding what you need to buy before you go. Your VIP can't always work out what he has in his cupboard because he can't distinguish all the jars and tins from each other.

The penfriend records your voice and creates a scannable label based on what you've said. It requires training and discipline to use effectively, but once conquered it is very helpful.

You speak into the penfriend as if it was a microphone. It then creates a small coloured label that can be attached to whatever you are labelling. The label has its own barcode so that when you scan it back, you will hear the message you recorded via the penfriend.

This device has multiple uses. Your VIP can label tins of soup, CD collections, DVDs, medicines, whatever he fancies. When he's out shopping, he can create a label for spaghetti hoops as he selects the tin, or else label it later. When he runs the scanner back over it, it will helpfully inform him, 'spaghetti hoops,' or 'Led Zepplin plays Barry Manilow'.

The penfriend can also be used on documentation to make items easier to find. Council tax bills, television licence – just pop a label on the top corner of each document.

Although the penfriend is a great piece of equipment, it needs to be introduced at the right time, when the VIP is ready for it. It requires work to keep it useful. Certain personality types, like me, would go 'Wow!' and label everything in sight for the first two days before forgetting about it. If your VIP was always very organised before his visual loss he is likely to love the penfriend.

Digital/computer devices

If your VIP is used to using computers, great; you can help him move on to new forms of computer use now that he's lost his vision. If, however, he has never used a computer before, this next series of tips may be too mighty a step for him.

You know your VIP and whether he is likely to be able to cope with certain technologies. Don't forget we are trying to reduce his overload rather than increase stress.

The buying, setting-up and installation of any computer device will need to be supervised. It is often beyond the wit of seeing adults to install routers, mobile phones or printers; with poor vision, such things are bewildering.

Once the set-up has been carried out, your VIP will need to be trained in how to use his new equipment. If you're less than confident with technology yourself, consider recruiting a 'technology coach' for your VIP. Often this will be a young person, preferably in their 20s or 30s.

You may have someone suitable in your own circle of family or friends – you don't need a computer engineer, just an average member of the public who is technology-literate.

Whoever it is, he will need to be able to explain things slowly and well because of all the jargon and new concepts. Some young people will explain the whole thing in 30 seconds flat, and assume that your VIP now knows what to do. *You need to select the technology coach with care. He will require patience.*

There is outside help available for computer device training. Contact your local library, Barclays Bank, your local Age Concern or Blind Association. They will all be able to help with training at the basic level, or they will know where to go for help if they can't work directly with your VIP.

Probably the most important device for VIPs

- Audio interfaces e.g. Amazon Echo/Google Home

Followed by:

- Tablet computers
- Mobile phones
- Synapptic software for mobile phones
- Computer keyboards for ease of use
- Supernova magnifier and speech software for use on an existing computer

There have been two devices that have been game changers for VIPs in my career, though neither have been specifically designed for VIPs. The first was the Apple iPad, but the most important is the Amazon Echo or Google Home.

Since the introduction of the iPhone, the pace of technological change has been astounding. However, VIPs have often struggled with these changes, as you need vision to use much of the new technology. The interface has always been some form of keypad that you have to see in order to use.

In this respect, the introduction of voice-operated computers is truly revolutionary.

The ability to use voice commands to operate a computer instantly opens up the world to a VIP. For instance, Amazon wants people to buy stuff from it as easily as possible, so it came up with the Amazon Echo device to make buying online simple.

An unintended consequence is that Amazon Echo makes life much better for VIPs. Initially your VIP may only use technology like this for a couple of tasks, but within a short time something like the Echo is likely to be an indispensable part of his life – which is what Amazon is after, of course.

As time passes new voice-operated apps will doubtless turn up. As coach, you will need to keep an eye out for these.

Of all the devices that are available and which you might consider buying, I would make either Amazon Echo or Google Home number one on your list (assuming the VIP already has computer experience). This is over and above virtually every other device for whatever purpose in this book.

Once your VIP is comfortable using the internet the world is his oyster. He can manage his banking, order food, arrange holidays, book taxis – in other words, almost everything that is available to someone with good vision.

In time he will also be able to operate white goods like washing machines, cookers, microwaves via Amazon Echo, Siri on Apple computers, Cortana on Microsoft, or Google Home. Control of additional devices isn't widely available as I write, but by the time you read this it will probably be different.

Tablet computers

The second most useful piece of kit that has emerged during my career is the tablet computer. The original Amazon Kindle and the Apple iPad were the first such examples, but these have since spawned a whole new generation of handheld devices.

If your VIP hasn't used a tablet before, the best idea is to let him try one out – perhaps your's, a friend's, or a family member's. Set up a session to show the VIP something that might interest him.

Tablet computers are so intuitive, you may be surprised how quickly they can be mastered by someone with poor vision. If you start your VIP off gently with a couple of tasks, it won't be long before he strays into new features and his confidence will blossom.

The original Kindle was an eBook reader. The most obvious benefit of switching to a tablet computer is that it may improve your VIP's ease of reading. Tablets have distinct advantages over conventional paper books if you have poor vision.

- The font size is easily changed, so you instantly have a large print book, whatever book you are reading.
- The weight of the tablet is the same whether it is in small or large font (whereas a big print book is very heavy, because larger print always results in more pages).
- A tablet is self-illuminated, so easy to see.
- The contrast can be switched so that you can either have black print on a white background or white print on a black background. Top tip: the conventional format for a book is black print on white paper, but if you go into 'Settings' on a Kindle or iPad you can reverse this. White print on a black background is often preferable for those with poor vision, as the print stands out better due to the higher contrast.

These are all significant advantages over old-fashioned print, but a tablet's usefulness does not stop there.

The original Kindle was effective at making reading easier. However, it has since become more than a reading device. Kindles are now full-blown computers, and along with Apple's iPad and Google's android devices, they offer some incredible opportunities to make life easier for your VIP.

Here are just some of the potential uses for your VIP's tablet computer:

- To translate type into spoken text
- To listen to emails
- As a magnifying glass, either directly in real time, or by using its camera to take a photo which your VIP can then magnify. A tablet's inbuilt camera creates a stabilised image that is not constantly moving - very useful for reading signs at a distance.

Please remember, though, that these devices won't give your VIP the pleasure of leisure reading. They are for functional reading (instructions, bills, letters, etc); if your VIP has lost significant vision, novels are probably never going to be possible again.

Mobile phones

If your VIP already has a mobile phone, a newer model may be useful for him. You can now buy models that talk back to you, or smartphones that have easy controls. The technology changes so rapidly, though, that I hesitate to recommend any particular models. This is an area where research is vital before buying. If your VIP has never used a mobile then the introduction has to be carefully planned. Allow plenty of time for training and play, or the phone may be quickly abandoned (or else mega bills may arrive in your VIP's name – neither option is desirable).

One product I will mention is the Synapptic app, which can be bought and installed on an existing android phone. (At the time of writing, there is not an Apple version.) This is a piece of software that will speak as you touch the keyboard/pad. There are other devices that also do this, but the clever bit about Synapptic is that it works in reverse on the keyboard/pad. If you touch a number when dialling, for instance, it doesn't dial the number until you remove your finger from the phone. This means if you touch a 5 rather than a 6 it won't dial the 5 automatically; simply slide your finger across to the 6, and when you lift your finger, it will dial correctly. This type of technology makes it much easier for your VIP to dial telephone numbers with confidence. Simple but clever. You can buy phones with this feature already installed direct from Synapptic (www.synapptic.com).

A lot of iPhones or equivalent can also be used as handheld magnifiers.

Software with computers

Another very useful piece of software is Supernova, which is available from www.irie-at.com. This is designed to blow up an image on a VDU screen to make it easier to see. It will also translate written text into audio so your VIP can listen to it.

There are specific text-reading machines available for blind people, often at high cost. Nowadays, software to adapt mainstream computers can be just as effective.

Further help with equipment

For an idea of other equipment available, search for 'low visual aid devices' or 'low visual aid magnifiers' on the internet. It will bring up a host of organisations and firms willing to help.

A word of warning: catalogues for the blind and partially sighted can be the equivalent of one of those gadget magazines that come with the Sunday papers. It's so tempting to get 'stuff,' partly to show you are trying to help and partly because 'it might be useful someday'.

It is so easy to be seduced by advertisements for devices that sound wonderful and that promise an easier way of doing things, but caveat emptor applies. I have come across people who have spent thousands of pounds on items that have rapidly become white elephants hiding in the corners of rooms.

There is a young man, Gus, whom I see regularly; he has reduced vision due to albinism, and he is a great sounding-board for the devices that turn up every now and again. Whenever I get excited about some new bit of kit and show it to Gus, I'm met with a teenage grunt: 'I can do that on my iPhone'. The new bit of technology, often costing hundreds of pounds, is dismissed within seconds, and he is right.

One of the main problems with products for the visually impaired is the cost of specialised equipment. Products can be expensive due to their limited market and sophistication.

Mass-market goods have low prices due to low manufacturing costs. Facilities for VIPs are secondary to the main use of the device, so the goods remain relatively cheap, even if a VIP can in fact make use of them.

With any new technological device, you will need to try before you buy. This rule applies whether it is a standard device or a specialised piece of equipment for the visually impaired.

You should be able to find a local charity/organisation that holds a stock of kit for the visually impaired. Take a trip along to see what they have. They may be able to supply you directly, or they may loan or hire out equipment for you to try.

Exhibitions/roadshows

There has been such an explosion of digital devices over the past ten years that it can be difficult to keep up with the latest developments. A good idea, therefore, is to go to an exhibition for the blind or partially sighted, as new products are constantly appearing.

An exhibition is useful for several reasons. Being in an environment surrounded by people with similar problems is itself reassuring. It makes a VIP aware that there are many people out there with visual loss. He realises he is not alone.

There are many exhibitions for VIPs held around the country. The major suppliers of equipment will be at the bigger shows. If you live in a rural location you may find a local event, but it is likely to have a limited number of exhibitors. The main regional cities have regular shows.

Sight Village, for instance, holds roadshows in London, Birmingham, Glasgow, Edinburgh and Manchester. Look on its website for information. These roadshows will attract all the major manufacturers. You may attend because you are looking for a specific piece of equipment, but you are likely to discover all sorts of other equipment, organisations and advice. A visit will never be wasted time, but it will most likely be an exhausting experience for your VIP, so be sure to plan it carefully to conserve his energy.

A company worth mentioning is Independent Vision (www.independentvision.org.uk). It hires out equipment on a monthly basis. It has a fairly wide range of equipment, from electronic magnifiers to text-reading machines. If you hire the equipment and then decide to buy it, your hire fees will be subtracted from the price, which is a good solution for both sides. (This hire offer is only for bits of kit worth thousands of pounds, and not small items.)

KEY POINTS

- If your VIP has ever used a computer, buy an Amazon Echo/ Google Home – the most important device now available
- There is a lot of helpful equipment out there. Use Google to search for examples
- A local support group is a good source of information about where to get stuff, which suppliers to use, what works and what doesn't, but don't be too influenced by individual views (one man's meat is another man's poison)
- Look at the RNIB shop online: www.shop.rnib.org.uk
- Visit www.abilitynet.org.uk for advice, ideas and equipment
- A specialist supplier of adapted equipment is https://www.cobolt.co.uk/
- Attend an LVA exhibition if possible. Check first with your local blind association
- You need a technology trainer for your VIP – a friend, family member or acquaintance who will make sure he can use and understand his equipment. Patience and technological knowledge are crucial requirements.
- Above all, look before you leap with any tech kit

I don't mind making jokes, but
I don't want to look like one

– Marilyn Monroe

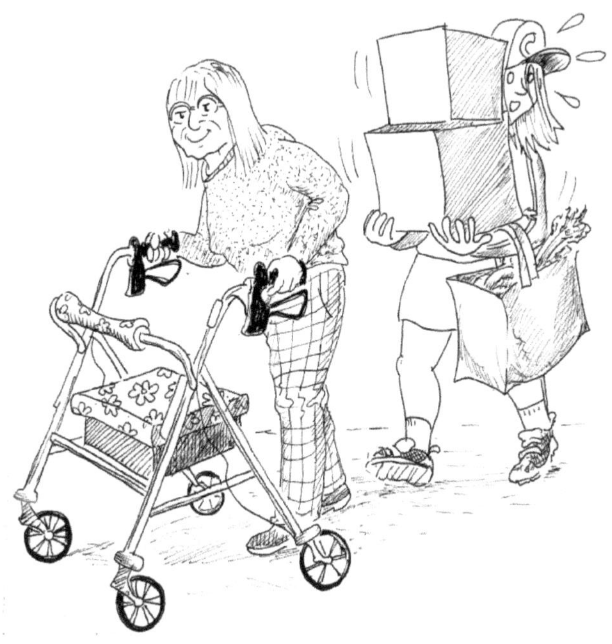

CHAPTER 15

Personal Presentation And Grooming

In our quest for an independent VIP, we have to deal with the subconscious fears that undermine her and of which she may be barely aware. One of these is confidence in her appearance and behaviour in public, particularly while she's eating. Mastering these fears is a crucial building block in getting your VIP back out in the world.

The way we are viewed is the result of a combination of factors cultivated over our lifetime. It's not that we are vain, but we all have a personal image that is just 'us.'

From our hair to our shoes, we all have a 'look'. Women have their favourite makeup, while men choose whether to shave or not. We wear clean clothes, whether our style is high-fashion or the 'unmade bed look'. It is critical to our self-esteem that when we appear in public, we appear as 'us'.

Imagine discovering that you have been shopping in a mismatched outfit that is dirty and covered in breakfast, with your hair all over the place. You may have had a conversation with a neighbour or friend who may not have commented on your appearance, though they will certainly have noticed it.

This is the reality of day-to-day life for the VIP.

Getting dressed

We dealt with decluttering clothing in the Home chapter, and discussed how the selection of clothing day-to-day can present problems for your VIP.

Organisation from toe to top is the answer.

Shoes should be kept in pairs. Organisers/hanging pouches are ideal. You might consider putting the most formal at the top and dirty old ones at the bottom.

Women might choose to separate shoes by colour or degree of fashion.

Socks should be kept together. Tights or stockings could be separated by denier. You may wish to check tights/stockings regularly for your VIP in case they are laddered.

Underwear isn't a problem for men, normally, but women may need a series of drawers, bags and baskets for different uses, colours etc.

Your VIP's main problem with dressing, though, is the outer, visible layer that the world will see. As coach, you need to find a way sort her wardrobe so that she doesn't go out in a horrible clashing set of clothes.

What you need is a brainstorming session, in which you decide on a system that is easy to use and remembered by your VIP.

Perhaps sort things into matching outfits – tops and bottoms – and then put a label in the same place on all trousers, shirts or blouses that might work together.

Consider a different label on colour-match sets, whatever kind of label the VIP can easily distinguish by sight or feel. (You could use a small safety pin for the first sets, two pins for the second set, three for the third set, etc – or whatever system works for your VIP).

Personal care

Having decided what to wear, a critical consideration is whether the clothes are clean. One area that is particularly difficult for VIPs is 'spotting.' We all drop spots of stuff down our fronts, or leave bits of shaving foam on our ears, or look in the mirror to see lipstick on our teeth.

The VIP will need someone to check her out before she appears in public, someone who can quietly let her know she has spinach trapped in her teeth or on her clothes. This task must be delegated to someone she trusts.

Very often it is the act of getting ready that creates 'spots' on clothing. Cleaning your teeth, shaving, looking after nails, putting on makeup; with a little thought, and perhaps a change in behaviour, most of these accidents can be easily avoided.

One couple I met told me that the husband struggled with shaving now that he couldn't see. This surprised me, as I have never looked at myself when shaving.

This may be too much information, but I have always shaved in the shower. I shave by touch. I never look at myself when shaving. Having used my razor, I feel the area where the blade has been, and if it is still stubbly I shave again.

This goes back to our habitual behaviour. I don't look at myself while shaving. The gentleman I just mentioned felt he must see in order to shave. Neither way of shaving is correct – they are just habitual ways of doing a job. If you have always stood in front of a mirror, the idea that the mirror is a vital component is hard to resist.

I also never use shaving foam or cream, so I never get white patches hanging around my face. This can happen all too easily with foam, and can be difficult to get rid of.

Teeth cleaning can also be messy. The problem is getting the toothpaste only in your mouth. Some VIPs bypass the toothbrush; they put the toothpaste on their finger, then in their mouth. This avoids the danger of dropping it in the sink or on clothing. Having cleaned her teeth, the VIP might want to consider washing her face to ensure she has removed all traces of toothpaste.

In the morning, it may be easier for her to clean her teeth before dressing – no toothpaste-decorated clothing.

While we're on the subject of grooming, nails can be filed with emery boards or trimmed with clippers rather than scissors. The emery boards will avoid all danger of nicking the skin and causing bleeding.

Now, hair. We all have bad hair days (every day for me). Poor vision can be particularly challenging for women in this respect, as they tend to have more elaborate hairstyles than men. Particularly if your VIP is female, her hairstyle may need to be modified so that it can be more easily maintained each day. Her sense of touch, though, is invaluable when it comes to managing her 'look.' Discuss with a hairdresser how to create a manageable style for your VIP.

Makeup

Many women are unhappy about going out without some form of makeup. It can give that much-needed boost when appearing in public, but it can also be a double-edged sword. If applied badly – and if this 'failure' is mentioned in public – it might prove devastating for your VIP.

This is one area where 'play' exercises are very useful. There are some great videos on YouTube that tackle the business of applying makeup if you are blind or partially sighted. Use these with your VIP as a means of problem-solving. The videos are mostly made by visually-impaired teenagers. These teenagers have tackled the problems that arise with makeup application and have found solutions. Their videos are informative and fun to 'watch' and listen to. Google 'Assistance with makeup when blind' for more information. (Isn't it ironic that you have to watch a video made by a blind person for another blind person?)

Bathrooms/bedrooms

I apologise if I sound like a cracked record, but so many aspects of personal care come down to the organisation. Your VIP needs to be able to find what she wants when she needs it.

Health, hygiene and personal grooming are often dealt with in the bathroom. Medicines, washing products and makeup usually jostle for room around the sink area.

In an ordinary bathroom, the toothpaste may lie alongside a haemorrhoid preparation cream or a tube of cosmetics. All have their specialist use, but they're decidedly not interchangeable.

In an ordinary bathroom, there is little fear of mistaking these products for something else. Now, in your VIP's bathroom, there is very good reason to separate them (keeping personal products in the bathroom, perhaps, and makeup in the bedroom).

Health care and medicines should be moved to a more appropriate place. Your VIP certainly doesn't want to confuse them with other tubes, tubs or packets.

Laundry

Having clean, fresh clothes is a confidence booster. Your VIP's whole laundry routine is another area that is suitable for a play exercise.

Does your VIP need to relearn the washing machine controls, or to get a new machine with a simpler control panel?

When buying washing powder, I recommend switching to a tablet or capsule system. It cuts down on mess and you always get the correct amount of powder.

Even for VIPs, it's easy to bung everything into the machine. The problem for those with poor vision is sorting clothes out, before and after washing. They need a system for sorting laundry, so they know they're washing the right things at the right temperature.

For the pre-wash sort, there are different systems your VIP might want to consider: by colour, if clothes are not colourfast, or by material. Colour is fairly easy for VIPs – simply divide into whites and non-whites, then wash all on a low-temperature wash.

Sorting for material is reasonably easy by touch, but some clothes can't be spun or tumble-dried. Your VIP may need two washing baskets, one for tumble drying and the other for non-tumbling. It seems excessive, but if you sew a little label into clothes of a particular characteristic (texture, colour or size), it makes it easy for your VIP to know what to do with it when it comes to laundry day. This avoids the danger of shrinking a much-loved top down to a child's size.

Post-washing, the main niggle (regardless of vision) tends to be matching up socks. But I have the ideal solution: ensure all socks are exactly the same. Throw away all variant types so that your VIP only has one style to manage. In theory, this is foolproof – but over time your VIP will need new socks, and you'll discover it's impossible to find the same style and colour again, and before you know it you're back to mismatched socks.

Some people try to pin socks together when washing to keep them as a pair. My wife forbade me trying this as an experiment, on the grounds that the washing machine was new. She didn't want it broken, and she thought the pins would tear the socks. Over to you on that experiment!

Internal labels of the sort you stitch in can also be used for sorting when you want to store items in drawers or cupboards.

Ironing

Ironing clothes is best avoided by switching to iron-free garments. When your VIP's clothes need replacing, buy easy-care items. Over time, most items can then be worn without the need for ironing.

An iron is a potential safety hazard. If your VIP insists on ironing, ensure she:

- Makes sure the settings are marked in a way that can be identified.
- Sets the temperature with the iron cold.
- Fills the cold iron with water using a funnel.
- Uses an ironing board, but places the iron on a heatproof worktop surface beside the board. The worktop should be large enough and clear of other items, so that the iron is easy to pick up and put down when hot.
- Wears a light glove on the hand to protect from burning if she touches the iron.
- When reaching for the iron, she should not reach for it directly. Instead, ensure she runs her hand up the flex to find it. She will feel the tension in the flex as she nears the iron and the heat.
- Ironing is one of those tasks which can be done very efficiently by feel. The VIP will feel the wrinkles in the cloth. She should stretch the cloth out on the ironing board to run the iron over it again.
- Ensure she practises all the above with a cold iron first.

Eating in public

It's the details of life that can trip one up. They are not big things, but they are the base blocks of living.

We take little things for granted when we can see. One such thing is eating.

We have already discussed 'toddler syndrome' and we all know the mess a toddler can make when eating. Your VIP will be painfully aware of this. We have all seen politicians make fools of themselves eating bacon rolls and bananas in public.

If you take your VIP out for a meal you will probably soon realise that spaghetti was not a good idea. Next time you have a meal, try closing your eyes before it arrives on the table. Try eating without looking.

A steak? In sauce? Big chips? Small chips? Peas? Now where did someone put that tall elegant wine glass with the long stem? Oh, you are wearing your best white outfit? And you've ordered a red wine sauce? Fine dining is a fiddly business. They put so much cutlery on the table, and the waiter has just warned you the plate is very hot.

If your VIP can read the menu (which is unlikely) it will not necessarily help with the confusing business of eating out. Simply picking a sandwich is not always straightforward. A chicken sandwich, for instance, sounds safe – but it may come as an open sandwich, or a huge stuffed roll with lots of extras dripping out of it, when an easy-to-eat, two-slices-of-bread-with-ham set-up was what she was hoping for.

For these reasons, and more, your offer to take your VIP out for a meal may not be greeted enthusiastically.

Cafeteria-style eating is difficult, too, for all sorts of reasons. The VIP can't see what she is ordering, so will have to ask what everything is. She will have difficulty loading a tray and then putting it down safely. If you are going to eat out, it is better to opt for a place with table service.

But we are getting ahead of ourselves. First we need to make sure the VIP can cope at home. Eating is one of those basic aspects of your VIP's life that has to be dealt with using tact and discretion. It is all too easy to humiliate the VIP with a word or phrase. Humour can help but it is a dangerous tool – you should always be laughing with them and not at them.

Hilda's story

Hilda had always prided herself on being well turned-out. She was a very feminine woman and was married to Fred, a retired bank manager. She was also, it must be said, slightly vain, and never went out without full makeup and good clothes – not even to the shops.

When Hilda lost her sight, she retreated into herself, to the extent that she wouldn't even eat with Fred at home. She still cooked, but Fred ate in the dining room, she in the kitchen. Hilda couldn't bear the thought of him watching her eat, of making a mess or not being ladylike in her eating habits.

Gently, Fred and I reminded her that her children had developed from their toddler eating habits to civilised ones, but that this hadn't happened overnight. They'd learnt how to eat politely with **practice**, and with 'feedback' (probably the wrong word) from her and Fred.

Hilda and Fred just needed to have a play around with technique. They hit upon the solution that Fred would cut up her food for her. Hilda learned to circle the plate from the outside in to get to the food.

Eventually Hilda began to eat out. They had always loved good restaurants. Fred would phone ahead and explain their situation, and the restaurant would cut up Hilda's food in the kitchen before serving. If the restaurant wouldn't help, they didn't get Hilda's patronage. She became quite relaxed about eating out eventually, even when minor mishaps occurred.

It can take several years to train a real toddler to eat like an adult. They have to learn a lot of skills. Your VIP has a head start here, but still, there are various new rules she may have to learn before she feels comfortable at the dinner table.

1. Gently investigate the table by hand to discover what cutlery is there.
2. When reaching for something (a glass or condiments) keep the hand low, fingers curved, and move slowly.
3. Ask for a sharp knife.
4. Check the balance of the knife/fork to judge the weight of food.
5. Ask for vegetables, salad or chips to be served separately and in a bowl, not on a plate.
6. Get food pre-cut before it arrives at the table.
7. To find food on a plate, circle in from the rim of the plate with a fork to the centre.
8. A bread roll can act as a buffer against which to push food if uncertain.
9. At a social event where people are standing to eat, ask for a seated position to avoid accidents.
10. Make sure the waiting staff understand about the VIP's sight on entering the restaurant (you may wish to do this on your own and in advance to avoid embarrassing the VIP).

Eating out alone presents more challenges for the VIP, mainly due to loss of non-verbal communications. How do you attract a waiter's attention to ask for water, coffee, or the bill when you can't see him?

The answer is simple: you discuss with the staff, either before you arrive, by phone, or at the time of arrival why you need that little bit of extra attention. Your VIP will usually get superb attention from caring staff. If not – well, that is the last time she need visit that particular establishment.

Personal care is an area in which we tend to be reluctant to interfere. Everybody has their own private habits and behaviours. However, in our quest for independence and an easier life for the VIP, it is something worth reviewing. Go over this chapter with your VIP, if only to stimulate conversation.

KEY POINTS

- Organise clothing for easy selection
- Review personal grooming routines
- Review laundry routines
- Practise ironing technique
- Discuss eating techniques and consider some pre-planning if you are hoping to go out for a meal with your VIP

Walking is man's best medicine

– Hippocrates

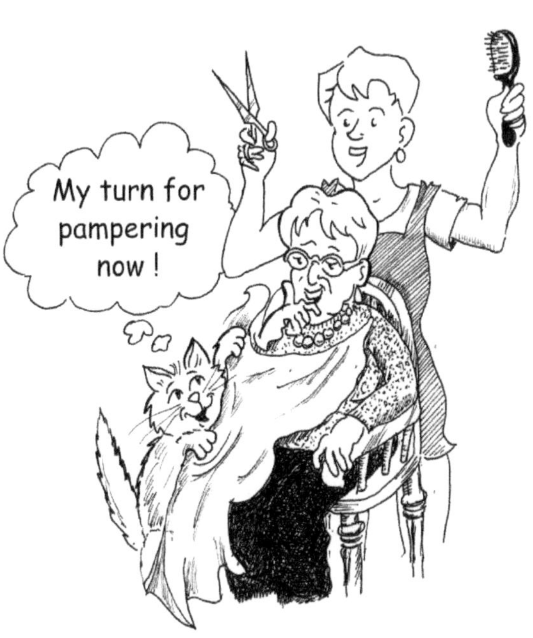

CHAPTER 16

Getting About Part 1: On Foot

Being independent is critical for your VIP's self-esteem and confidence. Going where you want, when you want is the main aspect of adulthood that a child craves. Visual loss can knock the VIP in so many ways, but feeling trapped in his own home can be the hardest blow of all.

The first, most fundamental form of travel I'd like to discuss is walking. All journeys require a few steps. We walk for pleasure and for a purpose, whether it be a stroll on a summer's day, or an essential journey to the dentist.

The action of walking itself is essential. The body and brain need exercise to work properly. Walking also stimulates by creating chances for social interaction.

So what is happening to make walking more difficult for your VIP, and how can we deal with these difficulties? Remember, the VIP has navigational vision but no detail. He can recognise the general street-scape: the outline of buildings, roads, where the traffic is, where people are. He should be able to walk around and not get lost without a problem.

The loss of detail is what makes walking difficult for him. He can't recognise people or pick out trip hazards like kerbs. Crossing roads is difficult; he will be able see an articulated lorry or a double-decker bus, but not judge how fast it is going or whether it is turning left or right.

Have I got time to get across the road? What is that driver likely to do? The small mental adjustments we make without thought are now difficult for the VIP. Cyclists are a nightmare, too, being small, fast and silent.

The VIP knows his neighbourhood and where he wants to go to. He will have an internal map of the area; he knows how to get to somewhere, and if there is a problem with his route he will be used to consulting the map in his head and adjusting accordingly. We all do this without thinking about it.

The problem with the map in the VIP's head is that it is a 'visual' one. He can 'picture' the layout of his town. What he needs now is a 'tactile' map of the town to overlay the original.

(As an aside, I would recommend you read the novel *All The Light We Cannot See* by Anthony Doerr[6]. It is about a blind girl in wartime France, and how she copes. It is a very good read on several levels, and will illustrate for you how a blind person orientates himself in order to get around.)

To create a tactile map of your VIP's area, he will have to re-learn his neighbourhood. Then he will be able to walk around safely.

As coach, this is where you come in. We are trying to build up the VIP's confidence so he can get out alone. The aim is to create a library of routes that he can use to walk to wherever it is he wants to go.

---

6 Antony Doerr. *All the Light We Cannot See* (2014) Scribner. ISBN 978-1-4767-4658-6

The simplest way to do this is just to go for a walk, turning either left or right from the VIP's front door.

It may be that your VIP will only use this 'library' to get into a taxi, car or bus. But he still has to learn how to get outside safely. This exercise should be used to identify any hazards that may cause him problems: steps, edges of pavements, drains, anything that is likely to cause a fall.

Note where the dropped curbs are ('Six paces after the lamppost, in front of the dry cleaners'). Find the safest crossing points if no pedestrian crossings are available. Look for any potential hazards or ways to make his walk easier.

It's your job to point out everything for him on the first walk. You can then repeat the walk as often as needed, until he knows where the hazards are without you telling him. Your VIP will eventually know the safest routes and will be able to walk through the neighbourhood on his own with confidence and competence.

You are building his new tactile map of the area. Eventually he should be able to tell you exactly how to avoid all the hazards as he goes. He will have learnt his route by heart and should feel confident walking about without your presence.

But don't try and learn the whole town in one morning. One route at a time is plenty as you build up different trips in his head. Practising the routes repeatedly is the best way to give the VIP the confidence to get about on his own.

Work with him on specific trips – the doctor's surgery, the chemist, the supermarket, the church hall, anywhere he goes regularly. For important places, like the doctors, practise going there even when he doesn't need to. The VIP may be stressed when he really wants to go to the doctor, which is when accidents happen.

Again, you are *playing*; concentrating on the process of getting somewhere and not on the goal of actually arriving. You are helping to build up your VIP's confidence and knowledge in a stress-free way. He needs to feel he can get around blindfolded.

By practising in this way, he will build up a series of new internal maps, so he can walk safely to wherever he needs to go. The 'tactile' maps will gradually converge with the 'visual' maps' in his head. It's a bit like a London taxi driver with 'the knowledge', constructing his own routes to get from A to B.

Having arrived at a destination, the next problem for the VIP is dealing with people when he gets there. We go places to do things – to go shopping, to get a prescription, to buy stamps at the post office, to have a cup of coffee; whatever it might be.

Two scenarios will illustrate some potential problems for the VIP.

Let's take a shop like Boots. The VIP can walk there on his own now that he has a tactile map of the neighbourhood. Let's say his purpose is to buy toothpaste. This is when it starts getting difficult. He may find the toothpaste section (if it hasn't been moved). But finding the right brand and size packet is more problematic. Has he just chosen denture fixative, or a tube of mascara?

Second, let's take a social event, or a meeting with many people present. Having got there, your VIP will have no idea who is in the room as he can't recognise faces.

Allow me to digress briefly here.

I have used the Vaseline glasses exercise many times with carers. What has always struck me about it is that people will only wear them for a minute or so before taking them off or looking over the top of the lenses.

I soon realised they needed to take off the glasses to understand what I was saying!

We have all heard that non-verbal communication is important. Supposedly 93% of communication is non-verbal and only 7% verbal. The non-verbal component is made up of body language (55%) and tone of voice (38%).

Michael Argyle, in his book *Bodily Communication*[7], says that a playful wink tends to be more effective than a well-thought out pick-up line. Non-verbal communication expresses emotion, supports words, reflects personality and underlies rituals such as greetings and goodbyes.

Non-verbal communications include gestures, facial expressions, eye contact and posture. Touch is non-verbal communication; a warm hug or firm handshake are quite different from a gentle pat on the back or a limp handshake.

Losing non-verbal communication is a neglected, unacknowledged facet of losing vision. Imagine going into a busy bar and trying to order a drink. It is difficult enough to attract the barman's attention when you have good vision. With no detail vision, you might find yourself wondering *are the people at the bar just having a drink or are they also trying to get served? Who is first in the queue?* We automatically take note of what is going on around us when we can see, and we follow a set of unspoken rules about being served. The VIP at the bar will be barging into a situation which is very tricky to read without those non-verbal cues.

People use non-verbal signals all the time. We may make a hand gesture to let somebody pass us. We smile to indicate we have seen someone. These communications often happen with no thought, but they help the world run smoothly.

Such signals go unnoticed by the VIP. Meanwhile, if he tries to convey information in the same way, he doesn't know whether the person has noticed it, as he can't see the reciprocal smile or hand movement.

This is when one of the biggest psychological stumbling blocks with loss of sight can rear its head. The VIP needs help, but he is reluctant to ask for it.

This reluctance is due to a combination of factors:

- Vanity
- Denial (not wanting to accept his handicap)

---

7 Michael Argyle. *Bodily Communication*. Routledge; 2 edition (3 Mar. 1988)ISBN 9780416381504

- His pride in being able to cope
- Not wanting to appear weak or vulnerable

These factors are understandable and real. All VIPs will experience them in varying degrees. Remember, they have slipped down Maslow's pyramid, so their self-esteem is at an all-time low. They may acknowledge this to themselves, but they certainly don't want to display it in public.

In short, they feel inadequate and miserable. In my letter in Chapter 9 I suggested the use of a white stick. This can be like a red rag to a bull for some VIPs. In fact it can provoke a reaction of outrage; the average person really, really does not want the indignity of using a white stick.

The subject of a signal cane needs to be raised with tact. If your VIP has just lost his sight the suggestion will probably be dismissed outright; it may then be difficult to reintroduce the idea for quite a while.

The average Joe makes the assumption that a blind person needs a white stick to tap his way along the road. Many people who are blind ***do*** need a long white cane, because they have navigational blindness due to glaucoma or retinitis pigmentosa. They have no peripheral vision so are likely to walk into things. But this is not the case with MD. Your VIP has navigational vision. He does not need a stick to get around.

This is what causes so much resistance. The VIP knows full well he can get around without a white stick, and this makes him feel guilty or embarrassed about using one. He doesn't feel 'blind enough' to do so. He doesn't want to be challenged about why he is using one. He may think he is a fraud.

As I said in my letter, though, the use of a white cane by someone with MD is not for his benefit. It is for other people, to make life easier for everybody. It replaces the VIP's non-visual communication. A signal cane levels the playing field; people will subconsciously realise they have to talk to the VIP, as opposed to making gestures.

Now back to real life. The VIP needs to understand he is sending out mixed signals to the world. He can walk into the shop or meeting hall with no problem. He doesn't have a guide dog. There's no visible indication that there is anything wrong with him. The general public will assume he is 'normal.'

When the VIP asks where the shampoo is in Boots, the average person will become confused. *Why is he asking me that?*

'*The shampoo is right in front of you,*' he might reply, before walking off.

But the VIP is none the wiser. He doesn't know which brand is in front of him, or whether it's for dry hair, oily hair, or those with dandruff. He needs more information.

Later, at the checkout, when he is fiddling around in his purse or wallet, trying to pay, the people at the back of the queue won't understand what the holdup is.

At a social event, the VIP may walk past an old acquaintance or someone he knows casually. The VIP won't acknowledge them because he can't recognise them. The other person will feel slighted, justifiably. '*I've known him 20 years and he cut me dead'!* Family and close friends will know of the VIP's poor sight, of course, but others may not know or won't remember.

The use of the signal cane oils the wheels of civilisation. It is good manners to use one. It ensures everyone understands what is going on. The VIP will be painfully aware at all times that he can't see detail, but the public will have no idea. The signal cane is a way of using non-verbal communications to open up real conversations.

The white signal cane can be kept folded up and out of view most of the time, perhaps lurking at the bottom of a shopping bag. If your VIP has a problem, he can reach into the bag and get it out. Just holding it folded in the hand is normally enough to get attention. Nine times out of ten the VIP will not actually need to extend it to a full stick.

With a stick in view, If the VIP asks a passer-by to help him cross the road or find something in a shop, the person will understand and may well help. The odd member of the Great British public may still ignore him, but most will certainly help.

When your VIP has experienced a few tricky situations out and about, he will begin to appreciate the benefits of the cane. He can ask questions which would appear foolish if he didn't have the signal cane in his hand.

Again, don't take on the battle about signal canes too early. It is often best to get the suggestion from a professional first, though you may need to nudge the professional to suggest it. Signal canes are available from the RNIB shop online.

Interacting with the public is often one of the main barriers preventing the VIP from getting out with confidence. The white stick is the way to unlock this problem. The VIP will know he has a problem in public, but most won't realise it is the loss of non-verbal communications that is causing him so much trouble.

Without a white stick, he is going to be like the wallflower at the party, ignored and in the corner, because the seeing world does not realise he can't communicate. If you don't know which person is the waitress, or the host, who do you speak to amongst all the people in a room? The VIP is going to feel unloved and unwanted at social gatherings if people think he has normal vision.

There are a couple of further topics to consider when it comes to getting your VIP out of the house.

Members of the public often assume all blind people own a guide dog. Most VIPs with MD can navigate safely on their own, however. They are unlikely to need a guide dog. In certain cases, dogs ***can*** be useful and people with MD have done well with them. However, your VIP needs to have settled into his own condition for some time before lurching off to get a guide dog. A call to Guide Dogs for the Blind is not a first step I would recommend in the rehabilitation of someone with MD.

On the subject of dogs generally, I like dogs and VIPs. A dog needs to be walked. It will make that need known. Taking a dog for a walk is great exercise and builds confidence. Dogs are a wonderful way to socialise with people. Dog owners always have an excuse to chat with each other. And who doesn't want to be loved unconditionally?

I certainly wouldn't suggest getting a dog, though, if your VIP has never had one. If he used to have one it ***may*** be an idea to think about getting one again. But it may create problems introducing a dog in the early days of a diagnosis. I would suggest that a dog is an idea for the longer term.

Mobility scooters are now in widespread use and can be helpful for those with MD. The general public regard visually impaired people on mobility scooters with a combination of humour and alarm; most don't understand the type of visual loss associated with MD, and so think their use is impossible. It is perfectly possible to use a mobility scooter with MD, however, though obviously a scooter needs to be used carefully for the safety of everybody. Your VIP certainly won't want a fast one and it cannot be allowed on a public highway.

On pavements, scooters are permissible for VIPs as long as due care and attention is taken. They are an effective way of getting around if used cautiously and slowly. Getting off or on one while brandishing a white stick is not diplomatic; your VIP may be unlucky enough to get abuse from the general public if he tries it, but for careful planned journeys on appropriate routes mobility scooters may be ideal.

The same applies for mobility scooters as for walking: you need to help him build up towards routes that are safe and navigable, with no tree roots, and with drop curbs, etc.

Your VIP's location

The final question for this chapter is the elephant in the room.

Is the VIP living in the right place? What may have been an ideal place to live with vision may be less than ideal now that he has poor vision.

Often in retirement, people move to a home that has been their lifelong dream. An uninhabited Scottish island, a cottage deep up a country lane; it may be idyllic when they move, but with poor vision your VIP's dream could quickly become a nightmare.

Your VIP may need to use public transport. Is it available? How much does it cost? How often is it available?

The cost of transport for simple trips could become prohibitively expensive (a £10 taxi ride each morning to collect the daily paper, for example).

Although I would not advocate moving house soon after losing sight, it may be necessary in the longer term. I have practised in a rural area for 30 years and I have known people who came to hate their place of retirement. The countryside can be a lonely place for those with poor vision.

For VIPs, instead of a rural retreat, a cottage soon turns into a pretty, rose-covered prison. This is more extreme in a village setting, but even suburbs can trap people if there are no local facilities.

This is a big, strategic decision. There are many factors to be considered. Sight is just one component in the big picture of life.

While you are pondering whether a move is necessary, your VIP will still need to walk about in his neighbourhood, wherever he lives.

KEY POINTS

- Go out with your VIP and practise taking safe routes to local places
- Buy a signal cane to counter the loss of non-visual communications

The VIP will have lost self-esteem and confidence. This has to be rebuilt slowly and gently. None of us want to make fools of ourselves in public.

A couple of bad encounters with uncaring people can convince your VIP that he doesn't want to go out alone again. if you escort him, he not only learns safe routes, but also how to interact with people when he can't read body language.

We travel not to escape life, but
for life not to escape us

– Anonymous

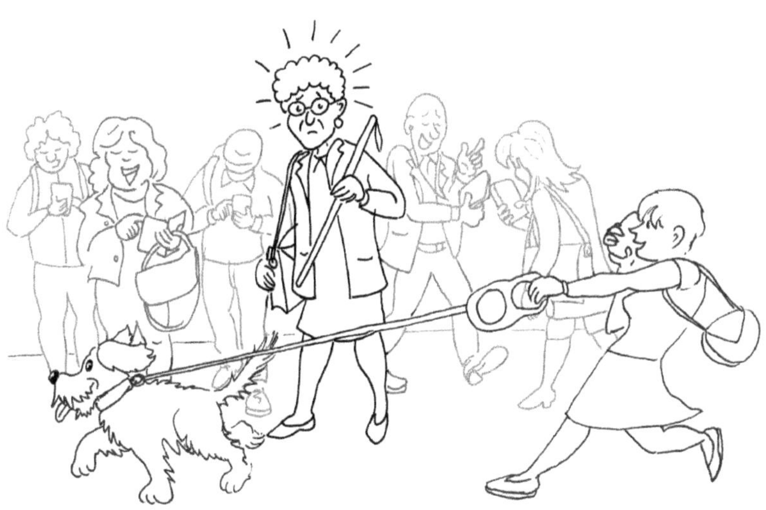

CHAPTER 17

Getting About Part 2: Public Transport

These days most lives are built around the car. Shopping, leisure activities, medical appointments, visiting family and friends: to lose a driving licence can be devastating. It is tantamount to chopping a person's legs off.

When you have access to a car, you spend little time planning or thinking about travel. You just go. With the onset of MD, though, journeys that can't be done on foot will change dramatically. Without a car you have to think so much more carefully about travel, be it by bus, train or taxi.

As coach, you have your own career or family to deal with. It won't be possible to do all the VIP's driving. It also may not be desirable. We are after all trying to maintain the VIP's independence.

If your VIP is living with someone who can drive this will be less of a problem, and if she has never driven you will just need to modify her existing arrangements.

There are two types of journey to consider:

- Local, regular journeys needing transport
- Irregular longer journeys needing public transport

Arranging a trip with less brain-processing power can be exhausting. Planning is required for even the simplest of journeys, and this workload is doubled when it comes to long-distance travel.

What routes are available? Where do you catch them? How often do they run? How do you get tickets? What firm do you use? Is it safe, is it clean, how do you get back...?

The first part of this chapter can be done from an armchair with a computer. It is an information-gathering exercise. Via Google, find out what is available locally for your VIP.

- Build up a personalised transport network for her. Where does she need to go, and when? Create a plan to get her there and back again.
- How is she going to travel? You will need to balance convenience against cost when deciding between bus, taxi and train.

Break down the details of each journey, bearing in mind that the available transport is unlikely to match the flexibility of a car.

- Your local county/city council sites will have comprehensive transport information, so look there first. Use search terms like '*(West Yorkshire) disabled transport*' and '*transport (South Somerset)*'. You will quickly get most of the information you need about your own area. It's amazing how much information is available once you start looking.

Once you have all the information, you have to match it up with what is needed by your VIP on a regular basis.

Some degree of negotiation may be required in terms of adjusting your VIP's timetable to the transport timetable. If she always went to town on a Friday morning to do the shopping (for instance) she may find she has to change to Thursday. If she always has coffee at a particular restaurant, it may be on the wrong side of town for the train, in which case a new coffee shop will need to be found. The bus may stop outside Morrison's rather than Asda, in which case a change of supermarket may be in order.

Learning a new supermarket or coffee shop will be difficult for your VIP in itself. Changing ingrained patterns of behaviour is challenging; if you change one thing you may find it has a cascade effect, and that this cascade then needs to be dealt with as well.

A degree of compromise is therefore in order. The VIP wants to live her life. You might regard some of her decisions as plain illogical. She probably thinks the same about some of your decisions.

A lady I know well insisted on visiting three different supermarkets. Each sold a particular item unavailable in the others. Trying to explain to her that other brands are available was met with a blank and pained expression. The phrase, 'You stupid boy,' was obviously going through her brain.

After the brainstorming/information-gathering session, you will need to go with your VIP during her first forays on public transport, especially if she hasn't travelled on buses or trains for years.

As with the walking exercise, she will be learning the routes and the hazards as you go. You can help with unexpected problems. More usefully, you are building her confidence in her ability to manage.

This, again, is the play stage. Process, not result, should be your aim. The most difficult aspect of negotiating public transport tends to be not the journey itself, but getting to the point of departure, and then getting from the drop-off point to the final destination. These can only be practised by doing real journeys. Until you actually do a trip, it is difficult to foresee what may go wrong.

Make it fun. Take journeys purely for pleasure. Visit a favourite place for nothing more than a stroll or a cup of coffee. If the first trip is a hospital visit, you have immediately ramped up the VIP's stress level. The whole trip is going to be traumatic. She won't be able to concentrate on the mechanics of the journey. She will associate travel with blood-pressure-inducing drama, to be avoided at all costs.

Sitting on the bus or train is the easy bit. As with walking, build up the routes: shopping, the doctor's surgery, the hospital, the bank, the church, the Women's Institute. All can be rehearsed and practised to ensure clear passage.

There are a lot of similarities between buses and trains but we will look at them separately.

Buses

The local authority website will contain all the basic information. In a way it makes life easy if there is only one bus suitable for where your VIP lives. In a city centre, transport will be more accessible for her, and simultaneously more complicated.

The local council website will explain any concessionary fares and the times they apply.

Payment methods are easier now in London and some big cities, with contactless cards and oyster cards widely available. Disability cards are also available in many locales. If possible, I would recommend organising payment before travel to reduce stress for VIPs.

Let's break down the stages of a potential bus journey your VIP may want to take (we'll assume you've already researched where she needs to go and how to get there).

She has rehearsed the trip to the bus stop.

She has arrived at the bus stop.

She is now standing there wondering when the next bus will be. Has she just missed it?

With real-time tracking of vehicles, you can find out when a bus is coming. Many bus stops have electronic displays to indicate which bus is next and when it should arrive.

Top tip

The LED display at a bus stop that shows information is often above head height. This is where the small monocular is invaluable. If your VIP brings it up to her eye she will often be able to read the display.

A monocular is about 3-4 inches in length and can be used quite discreetly. The VIP will then know which bus is arriving next and whether it is the right bus for her. This works well when it is a multiple bus stop, with buses heading to various destinations.

It your VIP finds it difficult to distinguish bus numbers as the bus approaches, the next piece of equipment to come into play is the symbol cane. If your VIP puts her arm out with the white stick then, legally, the bus should stop. It may be the wrong bus, but that doesn't matter. Your VIP should simply keep going until the correct one turns up.

Having eventually got on the right bus and having paid for the journey, all the VIP has to do is sit down and wait until the end of the journey.

Knowing when to get off the bus can be difficult, however. For those with normal vision it is easy enough to look out of the window, see the museum (or whatever you're looking for), and dismount the bus. Some buses have recorded messages that helpfully let you know that the next stop is the museum; this is helpful in principle, but such messages may not be available, or they might not be working.

You can still use vision as a prompt if this is a bus route that is likely to be used regularly. When trialling the route with your VIP, you'll need to work out some features beyond the bus that she can recognise. You'll need several different features, as we all drift off mentally at times. If your VIP can recognise the town hall, the tattoo parlour and the park, it won't matter if she stops paying attention for a few seconds; she will still recognise enough features to know she's reached her destination.

Again, this is where a monocular can be useful. You can use it to 'spy' features on the journey (though the bus does need to be stationary when using the monocular).

Asking for help can be problematic. Your VIP may inadvertently pick a non-local who has little idea himself of where things are. This, again, is where a signal cane is useful. It is a crucial form of non-verbal communication for your VIP, and others on the bus will at once understand why she needs help. Someone will almost certainly step in.

Bus travel discounts

If you are registered as blind or partially sighted, you can receive free or discounted travel on buses.

In England, your VIP can get an annual pass for free off-peak travel in her local area. In some areas, she might also be able to travel for free during peak hours. Contact her local council to find out more.

In London, she can travel for free all the time with a Freedom pass. The pass is provided by her London Borough Council.

In Scotland, your VIP and a companion can receive free local and national bus travel with a Scottish National Entitlement Card.

In Wales, she can travel for free at any time of day on local and national bus services.

In Northern Ireland, she may be able to get discounted or free travel using a SmartPass. Find out more with NI Direct.

In Liverpool, she may become a 'twirly'. Pensioners line up at the bus stop and halt the bus with the cry, 'Am I too early?' (They are not allowed to use the buses until 9.30am.)

To avoid her being a 'twirly', get her a disabled pass. It will allow her to travel at any time at the discounted price.

There are some useful videos online, made by the RNIB, which are worth playing to further illustrate what I've said above.

Planning your journey

http://www.youtube.com/watch?v=hRO-53fGEFQ

Getting on the bus

http://www.youtube.com/watch?v=_EhwZNuFQP4

On your journey

http://www.youtube.com/watch?v=I0xLWSpi5Kw

Getting off the bus

http://www.youtube.com/watch?v=0z1EqrqzaF4

Trains

The procedure for trains is broadly similar to buses. You'll need to look into times, routes and payment procedures in advance. The same research needs to be done and the same problems thought through before your VIP undertakes a journey.

Trains are used for longer, irregular journeys that are not likely to be repeated often. It may also be necessary for your VIP to change trains, and even to cross a city like London.

As with all these exercises, start at a simple level. If train travel is required, try out the simplest journey possible. You will need to work up to a mammoth cross-country trip.

The beauty of train travel is that you have clearly defined start and finish points. All stations have clear signage. The minus points can be finding the right platform, negotiating the train doors and minding the step on to and off the train from the platform.

Again, a monocular is invaluable, and is even more effective on railways. Your VIP can use it on the platform to read departure times and platform information. Once on the journey, every stop can be checked in this way, as all stations have big signs displaying place names clearly. There is also display information in most carriages now.

Another big advantage of train travel is that train companies have to accommodate people with disabilities. There is a comprehensive rail assistance system in place that can be accessed by your VIP.

All train operators across the UK provide travel assistance for people with sight loss or other disabilities. This usually includes guiding the VIP to the platform and meeting her at her destination. You can look online for information about assistance from your local operator, or go to the national websites. Type 'assistance for your journey' into Google. This will bring up information about national and local help.

If your VIP is going to need assistance to travel, contact the train operator in advance. Some operators offer a turn-up-and-go service, and at large busy stations help may be readily available; but it is better to be prepared, and at a country station you should always check before she travels.

This rail assistance service will offer help in getting on the right train, and then further assistance with onward travel once your VIP has reached her destination (this can include help getting to another platform or to a bus stop or taxi rank).

Ticket costs

Your VIP is eligible for discounts when travelling by train, depending on time of travel. You can also get discount for somebody travelling with the sight-impaired person. This is very useful and can encourage companions to go along for the trip. Contact train operators for more information. There are blind tickets available, as well as the Disabled Persons Railcard. It is worth investigating which would be more useful. This, again, is an armchair exercise best done on a computer.

At the end of the journey, your VIP will need to get out of the station. She will then need to walk, or access another form of transport, to her destination. Repeated journeys will build up her 'muscle memory' for such journeys and will make travelling easier in future.

Brian's story

Brian has been a VIP for many years. He is a confident traveller, but he still gets caught out occasionally. On this occasion he was crossing London from Waterloo to Paddington, a trip he had done several times by underground. On this particular day there was an incident on the Bakerloo Line. Whilst at Waterloo, Brian heard an announcement telling him that the line was closed.

Like Luke Skywalker with his lightsabre, Brian unleashed his signal cane while he thought about the problem. Immediately a railway official appeared at his side and offered to help. He escorted Brian down to the correct platform and waited until the train arrived.

The official then informed the driver that he had a VIP on board. Brian got on the tube. The standard recording was played at every station, but the driver still made a special announcement for Brian to help him get off at the right place.

Another tube worker was waiting for Brian to take him to the next platform. He was personally escorted on every leg, all the way to the exit at Paddington. Brian said he really did feel like a VIP.

Taxis

Taxis are extremely useful and are the simplest way to go door to door. The main problem is expense.

Research is useful here. Taxi drivers are just members of the public. Some are rude and some are helpful; it is worth spending time investigating the local taxi firms. Some make it their selling point to cater for people with disabilities.

Try to find two or three drivers who are sympathetic and helpful when picking up and dropping off. If your VIP is on first name terms with a driver who knows her, travel is likely to be a much better experience.

With her new, easy-to-use mobile phone already set up, with the local taxi firm on speed dial, your VIP has a 24/7 chauffeur service at her fingertips, worthy of any self-respecting oligarch.

Local transport schemes

Local accessible transport schemes are many and varied. The place to look for these is on your local authority website under 'transport assistance (Devon) blind'. You may need to play with the searches a bit, but every area will have its own schemes.

There are 'dial-a-ride' or 'ring-a-ride' schemes where your VIP phones for a minibus to take her door to door. These usually need to be pre-booked. She may need to be registered for the scheme through the local authority.

For access to medical facilities, there are almost certainly local services available. These may be particular to the GP surgery, or maybe arranged via the local ambulance service for hospital visits. Again, time spent on the internet is invaluable. Keep your ears open to unearth special projects for all sorts of activities.

Again, you can visit the Sightline directory online (sightlinedirectory.org.uk) for useful information.

A particularly good service can be found here: rnib.org.uk/travelsupport

This support service can pair your VIP with a trained volunteer who will:

- Help to plan journeys, find timetable information, arrange assistance and buy tickets
- Accompany her on a journey she can already do, but which she would like to be more confident making on her own
- Take her on a new journey so she can learn the route

KEY POINTS

- With all forms of travel, advance planning takes time and trouble, but is well worth the effort. This applies from the simplest local walk to cross-country trips by public transport
- Travel is one of the areas where you may well need help getting it all done. It is also one of the few areas where it is relatively easy to access practical help for your VIP. The time spent organising trips could pay dividends in terms of giving her back confidence and independence
- Work slowly, route by route. Access the information in a form that can be used by someone with poor vision (for instance, large print or audio maps that can be carried with her, so she can get back home if she has to change plans)
- Learn the routes to and from the bus stops and train stations at both ends of the journey
- Explain about use of a symbol cane to stop buses or to signify help is needed
- Consider payment methods, if possible paying for each ticket in advance
- Make use of helpful equipment: a monocular telescope, a symbol cane, contactless payment cards or travel cards
- Delegate transport duties to somebody with the time and patience to help
- Visit rnib.org.uk/travelsupport for further information

Now we just need to deal with what to do when your VIP has got to her destination.

I went window shopping today!

I bought four windows

– Tommy Cooper

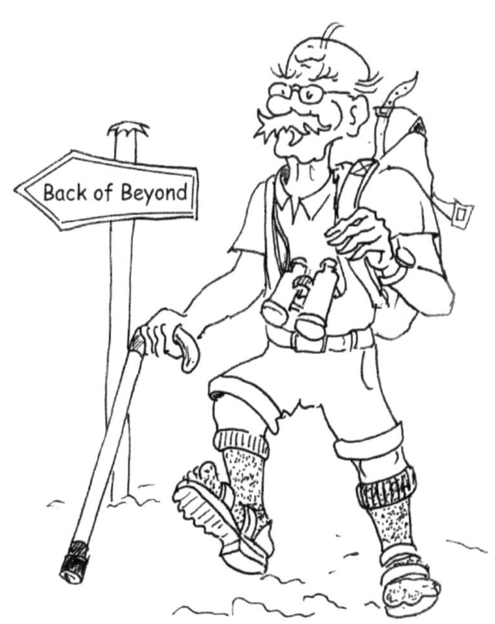

CHAPTER 18

Shopping

Paul's story

Sorry about this, but I'd like to tell you about my experience of going into a shop wearing Vaseline-covered glasses. I was on holiday with my sister, a bemused companion, having not wanted to embarrass myself locally.

It was a small farm shop/deli, with an assortment of chilled display cabinets. There were all sorts of delicious pies, pastries and salads laid out; just the produce you would expect to find.

I arrived in front of a glass counter that probably contained meat. There was an assistant/butcher on the other side. I guessed the produce was meat by the colour, but couldn't tell whether it was sausages, liver or prime steak. I had no idea what lay before me, being unable to pick things up to examine them.

The pies were a nightmare. They smelt great. They were clearly freshly cooked. To me, at a distance, they were just light brown blobs, and the labels were too far away to see. My sister had to tell me what everything was. I had no idea what was on display.

We reached the dessert counter, with cakes etc on display. Again, I had no idea what was there. My sister recited what was available. I selected a slice of banoffee pie.

We walked further around the shop. I felt a beer was in order and could make out some brown bottles. One beer being fairly similar to another, I was willing to take a risk on selecting one. We were on holiday after all. A local beer might be fun.

I picked a bottle at random and put it in the basket. My sister, in the way sisters do, plucked the bottle from my hands.

'You don't want that.' Miffed, I wondered why ever not. 'It's a chili-infused vinegar,' she retorted.

On getting to the checkout, I used the card machine. This entailed me picking the machine up and scrutinising it from about three inches away. I managed to stab the right numbers.

Later I discovered my banoffee pie was a major disappointment. Instead of a creamy slice of heaven, with soft toffee and banana on a pie crust, topped with whipped cream, I bit into a hard slice of biscuit-like a chocolate shortbread.

The lessons from my story are:

- VIPs can go shopping on their own, but there are limitations.
- If you have to rely on descriptions, you still may not end up with what you really want.
- If you can handle things, you're better able to work out what they are.
- You need to inspect goods carefully and not make assumptions.

Shopping as a VIP can be a bit like a blind date; you are not sure what you are going to end up with. With small purchases this may not matter so much, but bigger purchases could cause problems.

Loss of vision is going to change the VIP's shopping habits. This comes with a cost attached. Time, energy and brainpower will be necessary to sort out new strategies.

If your VIP previously used a car he may have shopped weekly, popping everything into the boot. Now, on foot or on public transport, he won't be able to carry much with him. He will have to get used to shopping more frequently. He may not be able to cope with heavy shopping at all.

One temptation can be to switch all shopping to the internet. While this is a very attractive idea, I would advise against it. The act of leaving home to go shopping is important in the wider context. Shopping gives your VIP a reason to leave the house. It is good exercise. He will meet and interact with other people.

Having to go shopping will keep him from retreating into a world 'home alone'. It will help rebuild his confidence.

For the purposes of this chapter I will treat 'shopping' as almost any commercial activity undertaken regularly. Food shopping, clothes shopping, hairdressing appointments, visits to cafés, the chemist, the butcher, the baker, the candlestick maker – you get the idea.

There are only two types of shop for a VIP

'Self-service' is meant to be an easy concept but, paradoxically, it is more difficult with poor vision than a place where you are served. Hairdressers, cafés, chemists (if the VIP is asking for a prescription) tend to be easier than the supermarket or clothing shops. The old-fashioned butcher, baker or candlestick maker are easier for VIPs, because you can ask for what you want.

We are so conditioned to modern shopping that this distinction passes most of us by, but it is useful to remember that small outlets often provide better service in this way for a VIP.

Using small shops or markets can also be helpful if more frequent shopping trips are needed because the VIP can't carry much.

The consequence of loss of detail and non-verbal communication has a further strange twist for VIPs. They will need to get used to communicating much more verbally.

If they go to the butcher's, for instance, they can no longer point and say, 'Can I have two of those, please?' Instead, they will have to ask what he has got in stock, how big the chops are, etc. This greater communication will create a deeper relationship with the butcher than you would usually expect.

The upside of this is that a VIP may truly begin to feel like a Very Important Person, with personalised service, rather than a Visually Impaired Person.

In a supermarket, or even a small store, as I experienced, it is almost impossible to go shopping without help if you are a VIP. The good news is that most supermarkets, with the exception of the deep discounters, will provide staff to help a disabled customer. The staff member will go around the store helping the VIP to find whatever he is looking for. Regular visits to the same supermarket will probably mean your VIP builds relationships with certain staff, but the bigger the supermarket the less likely this is to happen.

Lilly's story

Lilly came to see me and we were discussing how she was getting on. She had been diagnosed with MD and was now using a signal cane. She lived in town and was only a short distance away from the shops.

One day, on her way to the small local supermarket, she had to cross a busy road with fast-moving traffic. She was hesitant to cross as she was unsure of the traffic and its speed.

She decided that she would wait until someone came along to help her across the road. There were a couple of teenage lads hanging about, but she didn't fancy asking them. After a couple of minutes, though, no one else had turned up, so she approached the lads, signal cane in hand. She explained she couldn't see well and asked for help to get across the road.

One of the lads took her arm and escorted her across the road. As she went to go into the supermarket the lad held her arm a moment longer and asked if she wanted a hand getting home afterwards.

She told me she hesitated, but thought he was a nice lad and so she said, 'Yes, please.' She did her shopping, and when she came out the two lads had waited for her and they then took her home.

Lilly told me that this had changed her whole outlook. Now she deliberately asked for help when shopping. There were three reasons for this.

1. She got what she wanted and knew it was the right thing.

2. If she asked an assistant for help, he would get a break from shelf-filling for a couple of minutes, which they usually appreciated.
3. She realised that asking for help made the person she had asked feel good about himself. He had done something 'good.'

Lilly said that rather than causing confusion, she was bringing a little happiness into the world by asking for help. She now realised she wasn't a nuisance at all.

This is one of the upsides of visual loss – the making of new and deeper relationships than a normal customer would experience. These new relationships will also, with time, create trust. If the VIP asks for an opinion on some product, he will have confidence in any suggestions made.

Most people are creatures of habit. Your VIP will have his shops of choice, dating back to a time when he had good vision and may have driven there. Switching to walking or public transport may mean that the old shops are no longer within easy reach.

Finding a whole new set of shops is fine in theory, but here we come up against the defence mode of thinking. Why would the VIP want to change his habits? He likes the products at his normal set of shops and knows his way around.

As coach, little by little, you can wean him onto easier solutions. You will probably need to organise someone to help him on shopping trips initially. Any self-service store is going to mean he needs assistance. This may be someone who accompanies him or a member of staff from the store. Members of the public will help the VIP if he only wants a single item, but are unlikely to drop everything to escort him around for his full week's shop.

If the staff aren't helpful at the VIP's usual supermarket, change the supermarket. It's your VIP's money, after all. If the supermarket wants that money it will have to work for it by providing a service. Point this out to your VIP and try somewhere else with him. He may be delighted with a new store, but you may literally have to hold his hand the first time around.

Another defence mechanism for the VIP is simply to select stuff he always buys. With food shops, this can lead to a rather monotonous diet. It also falls apart when the supermarket rearranges the shelving. If your VIP relies on his memory to shop, his selection will quickly become limited.

If he gets help with his shopping from staff, there are two aspects to the relationship. The first is plain information. *Where do I find a packet of Hobnob biscuits? How much do they cost?* The second aspect is trust. *Do I trust their judgement? Will I like the meat lasagne they suggested? Have they picked out the most cost-effective product?*

If your VIP develops regular relationships with those who assist him at the shops, he is likely to receive suggestions for other items – perhaps a treat, a cheaper or more useful option, or a special offer. VIPs can be naturally fearful about trusting others to begin with, but these suggestions can be a real positive. Most shop staff will be pleased to be trusted by someone whom they understand is vulnerable, and they are unlikely to abuse that trust.

Communication and trust are at the heart of all trading situations. When your VIP trusts someone involved, and can chat to that person in a market, shop or supermarket, most of his problems will be solved.

Removing the VIP's fear of making a fool of himself is very important, too. We all cringe at the thought of being embarrassed publicly.

Paying for goods

Payment can present problems for VIPs. It may require a little thought and some advance planning. Handling cash can be difficult with poor vision;

wherever possible try to encourage your VIP to use bank cards, which saves him fiddling with notes and coins. For VIPs it is a good thing that we are rapidly heading towards a cashless society.

Most banks will supply credit or debit cards that have large symbols or a notch set in the surface, to help identify which way round the card is. Ask at the local branch for details.

If your VIP does need cash, go with him to his local ATM machine and have him practise using it. He will need to learn the keypad so he knows which way it is orientated. Normally the central button has a raised bump on it; it is then a question of remembering the pattern of his pin code movements from that central spot. Get him to try taking out £50 in £10 instalments one after the other as a practice. You will have earned a coffee between some of these practice sessions!

For VIPs, the easiest way to pay is via contactless payment cards, which involve simply waving the card over the card machine. Search for shops or cafés that use this system locally. Just going in and asking the question helps – the staff will happily explain how they can take your money in the easiest way. Again, this helps to build relationships with local traders. If staff are unhelpful, move on.

When using cash, your VIP will need to learn the different sizes of the notes. Get him to put a banknote between his fingers and measure it against the length of the finger. Each denomination will correspond to a particular finger size. The bigger the note, the higher the value. Along with the note's colour, this will enable the VIP to tell them apart.

For coins, a useful purchase is a money holder that sorts the coins by their different sizes.

A trivia point.

The blind American musician Ray Charles always insisted on being paid in single dollar bills. He was cheated early in his career by venues giving him single dollar bills rather than 20-dollar bills, dollar bills of all denominations are all the same size in the US. No matter the size of the payment with single dollars, nobody could cheat him.

Larger purchases

White goods, digital devices, financial products and clothing are different. They require judgement, while day-to-day supplies simply require help. For large purchases, your VIP may need the assistance of someone who is more clued-up on a given product.

So who is best placed to help your VIP? You are looking for someone who can be trusted to give good advice. With clothing, you are looking for someone who understands the person and what suits his style. You may need your tech team member for digital purchases, or a daughter for clothing advice.

With any shopping trip, the key is to keep it short and sweet. Remember the 'toddler syndrome'; you don't want to have a major falling out because your VIP is frustrated and exhausted.

Internet shopping

There is a place for internet shopping in your VIP's life. The internet is brilliant for bulky or heavy items, as they can be delivered direct to the VIP's door.

Initially, you may need to set up internet shopping for his groceries, from Ocado or Tesco, or whoever he wants to use. You can then pass it over to him once the shopping template is in place. The idea is that he should then be easily able to order stuff himself whenever he wants. Again, Amazon Echo or Google Home will be invaluable to him for internet shopping.

Labelling

A final problem with shopping. The VIP returns home with a bag full of groceries, having received excellent help from a staff member. But what is it all?

This is where some form of labelling system comes in. One simple example involves elastic bands. Put them around cans for your VIP – perhaps one for tomato soup, two for mushroom, or different coloured bands depending on the category of purchase. Any system which works for the VIP and can be remembered easily will be worth your time in the long run.

The easiest option is to label something as your VIP buys it. He then only has to identify it once. This is when a penfriend is most useful. Your VIP speaks to it, and it produces a label, which he then puts on his can of baked beans. The label can be scanned at home at a future date to help to identify what's in his cupboards. There's more information about the RNIB's penfriend device in Chapter 14 ('Technology').

Shopping is a really difficult task with poor vision, as I tried to illustrate with my fumblings in the farm shop.

Your VIP will certainly need help when shopping. This help will either have to come from the shops themselves or from another person. As coach, you are likely to need a 'team' member to look after his shopping.

You can do it yourself, of course, but it may be there is a better person available who is local to your VIP and who has the free time to be able to help. Finding that person is probably your most important task.

KEY POINTS

- You will need to sort out the VIP's route to the shops
- You will need to help him navigate his routes around the shop(s)
- Make contact with his regular shops, and find helpful individuals who are sympathetic to your VIP's situation. If staff are unhelpful, change shops
- Help him practise using ATM machines and handling cash
- Support him if he wishes to use internet shopping
- Consider a labelling system for goods
- Find a 'team' member to help with shopping

Don't walk behind me; I may not lead. Don't walk in front of me; I may not follow. Just walk beside me and be my friend

– Albert Camus

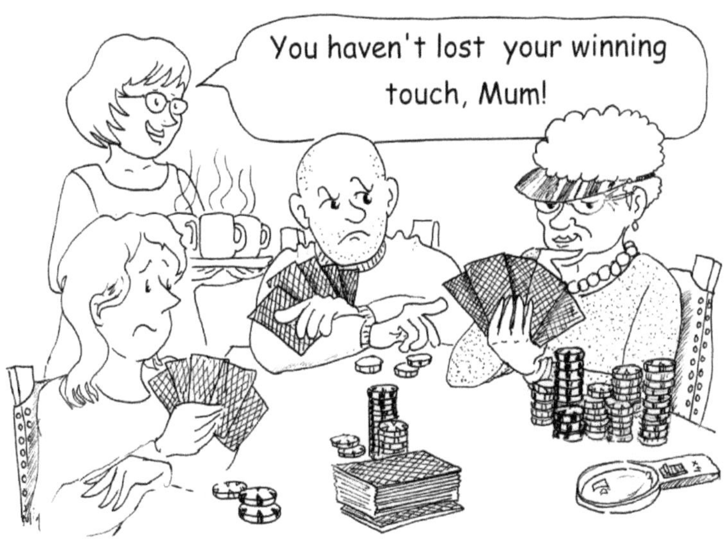

CHAPTER 19

Regaining A Social Life

Congratulations on getting this far. You are almost there.

You may have read to this point without necessarily having implemented anything. That's fine. You need an overview of the subject before starting out.

This chapter, though, is the goal you are trying to reach as your VIP's coach. The whole of this book has been in preparation for this topic.

At the outset, your VIP had slithered to the bottom of Maslow's pyramid. With the information, actions and ideas from the previous chapters, she will be back functioning at a basic level.

- She can live at home and use appliances
- She can feed herself
- She can get the information she needs
- She has technology to help her
- She can get around using different forms of transport
- She can cope with shopping

These are the foundations for living, and are wonderful achievements to have re-attained.

They are only foundations, however. Humans need friendship, intimacy and a sense of family. We want to feel a sense of belonging and acceptance. It is human to be part of a group, whether those groups are large or small.

The final hurdle for the VIP is to regain her social life. If she can achieve that, you will have managed to drag her back up Maslow's mountain to level three, where we should all be.

We are all members of diverse groups, from structured clubs like churches, professional organisations and sports teams, to non-structured groups, e.g. a bunch of friends who meet up occasionally.

On a small scale, our social connections are our family members, intimate partners, close friends and confidantes. These are the connections that make our lives by defining who we are. We need these relationships. Without a sense of belonging, without meeting people, we become susceptible to loneliness and social anxiety. This need for belonging is a powerful component of the human psyche.

If we fail to raise the VIP's confidence in getting out and about, she may 'shut down'. Serious health issues can develop if she becomes isolated. The immune system slows, making infections more likely. An almost literal death spiral can be created if your VIP loses her confidence in loving and being loved.

Relationship breakdowns can be a side effect of loss of vision. Family and friends may still profess to love her, but the VIP may feel unable to reciprocate. One-sided relationships are more liable to deteriorate. Either side may feel they can't make the effort any longer.

We need to get our VIP out and about and enjoying herself. As we've seen, though, loss of vision can make social situations difficult; the natural reaction for VIPs is to withdraw from society like a wounded animal crawling under a hedge for protection. Once this happens, it can be difficult to get them to re-engage with groups, friends, clubs, etc.

So how can you help?

You already understand the potential problems of social interaction for VIPs:

- Loss of non-verbal communications
- Social awkwardness associated with not recognising people
- Not being able to see to do tasks
- General exhaustion
- The difficulty of physically getting to places to attend events
- Ignorance about visual loss among members of the public

To rekindle a social life for your VIP, these issues need to be addressed.

It is so easy to get bogged down in the nitty gritty of daily life (sorting out transport, going shopping, hospital visits, paperwork) that social events may languish at the back of the queue.

The VIP may even feel guilty about asking you to arrange an 'outing' for her, and so never mention it.

This is why finding a 'social secretary' for your VIP is crucial – someone whose task it is to jolly her along and ease her passage back into taking part in events. You may even need an informal team to try and get her back on her feet socially.

A regular routine of social activities is what we are trying to achieve – preferably weekly events, as opposed to a random occasional coffee morning.

The ultimate aim is to get the VIP to attend events alone. She will almost certainly need support initially. Transport needs to be under control, for one; the VIP needs to feel comfortable in a venue and she has to be relaxed enough to mix in with the group, which means others at the event need to be comfortable with her.

She needs to feel safe, not vulnerable. When a child first attends school, its mum is prominent in the background to ease the transition. Your toddler VIP needs similar care to let her feel at ease again.

You also need a sense of what she used to do, what gives her satisfaction, pleasure and a sense of fulfilment.

- What, if anything, is she still managing to be involved with?
- What activities are limping along?
- What has she stopped doing?

You may know the answers to these questions immediately, but it is still worth putting on paper. Seeing it written down may give you a different insight. Going forwards, your VIP's main problems are likely to be:

1. How to get to and from each event.
2. How to reduce embarrassing social situations with a signal cane.
3. How to reduce some of her exhaustion, or to manage her time to limit fatigue.
4. You may need to discuss with those taking part in the activity the nature of the VIP's sight loss. Use the Vaseline glasses if necessary. If others understand your VIP's predicament, life will be easier for all.
5. Some new piece(s) of equipment may be needed to make it easier for your VIP to take part in a group.

There are all sorts of ways people might socialise, ranging from meeting a single friend for coffee to running an orchestra. Your VIP may have done certain activities all her life. Some interests may be more recent.

Whatever her particular interest, it should be possible for your VIP to continue in some form. It is remarkable how people can adapt to doing things in different ways.

Some social activities may be impossible for her to carry on with, however. If she was a look-out at the local coastguard station, or a fine embroidery enthusiast, she may need to think about a new hobby. No one expects to be playing five-a-side football at 70, or doing break dancing.

But this needn't mean a much-loved activity is now closed to her. Few organisations are willing to lose members or volunteers nowadays. Your VIP may be able to be re-deployed to another role. A trainer, an administrator, a tea maker, someone to man the phone – there are always jobs that can be done whether your VIP can see or not.

Changing roles in an organisation requires patience, and is not something to be attempted immediately after a loss of vision. Particularly if the loss has been quick, your VIP will need a period of adjustment before she can get back to a group.

If your VIP is willing to keep in touch with her established group, as time passes she can begin to identify a new role for herself. Some diplomatic liaison with the group may pay dividends. Then, gradually, when she has begun to cope with the basics of living, she can begin to take on new tasks in social situations.

Suggesting a completely new activity is not necessarily a bad idea, though. I would recommend either or both of the following:

1. A local self-help support group. The Macular?? Disease Society has local groups; they are rather haphazard, geographically, but attendance will provide your VIP with lots of support and information.

   Simply attending a self-help group will help her to realise that macular disease is a widespread issue. If she has had a problem, someone else at the group will have had exactly the same problem. They may also have suggestions for a solution.

   Just *listening* at this kind of meeting is invaluable as a way of learning how others cope. Conversations may throw up ideas that she has never thought of or considered.

   Most people tend to attend a self-help group for just a few months or meetings until they feel they have learnt enough to manage. If they feel altruistic, they may stay on to help the newer members who have joined more recently and are feeling lost and panic-stricken.

2. The 'Finding your Feet' courses run by Action for Blind will give the VIP the chance to ask questions and get answers on the spot (see Chapter 8 for more information). Self-help groups are more indirect; they are not manned by experts, though the attendees will probably know whom to ask locally for information.

Both of these are good starters for encouraging self-confidence in your VIP.

Sport

Lots of activities can be undertaken with MD. Just consider the 2012 Paralympics in London; it was awe-inspiring to see what can be achieved by people who are physically disabled. You may be surprised at the number of sports that can be done by the visually impaired.

A little digging will reveal what sports can be done by your VIP in the local area. This is where the local library and self-help groups come into their own. Buried deep in some file stuffed under a desk you may find some real gems of information.

Many charities and local groups work on tiny budgets, so are not well publicised, but they are always on the lookout for new members. They do brilliant work if only you can find them.

If your VIP has had an interest in sport all her life, this may be appropriate. A lot of sports have been adapted to allow for blind participants, so your VIP may be able to carry on almost as before.

In fact, if she has had experience of the sport before losing her sight, she can be extremely useful as a 'cross-over' – someone who previously played but is now blind. Cross-overs understand both sides of the sport. Non-blind helpers won't fully understand the problems of the visually impaired. A cross-over can act as a go- between for both sides.

My own sport, sailing, works well for blind people. The freedom of sailing a boat is often liberating for them. They can often 'feel' the boat better than many seeing people. They may just need a sighted person on-board for a few of the fiddly jobs.

I met a woman once who attended blind boxing training. She loved it; she got out all her frustration on a punch bag rather than on her husband.

Bowls is a game that has a well-organised blind league structure. I met a bowls player once who amused me. He came to get his vision assessed, as he played bowls in a blind league.

There are varying levels of disability for bowls. You play in an appropriate league depending on your standard of vision.

I realised after some time that this man really wanted me to classify him as more visually impaired than he actually was. He realised he would do better in a different league.

I had to admire his competitive spirit, but not his gamesmanship. He wasn't pleased when I failed to re-assign him. Just because someone has a disability it doesn't make him a better person!

On leisure activities

When my own mother was 83 she used to attend a botanical flower painting course. It was the highlight of her week, and she loved a good natter with the 'girls' on her course.

That course did more for her health than most of her trips to see a doctor. The stimulation of doing something she enjoyed, of learning a new skill, with friendly people around her, gave her a real focus to life, something to look forward to and dream about. The alternative is sitting in a morose puddle of depression and feeling that you have nothing to live for.

Dancing is a wonderful way to meet people and have fun. MD does not restrict either men or women from enjoying being held by someone, or from being whirled around a room to music.

Your VIP may appreciate a trip to the cinema. There are schemes whereby those who are registered blind or partially sighted can get a free cinema ticket for those accompanying them.

You need to sign up for a Cinema Exhibitor's Association (CEA) card. To apply for the card, you will need to prove that you receive a qualifying benefit: a Disability Living Allowance, Personal Independence Payment or Attendance Allowance. Alternatively, your VIP will need to be able to show that she is registered as blind (severely sight impaired).

For more information on how to apply and which cinemas take part in the scheme, you can visit the CEA card website or call 0845 123 1292.

Entry to places of interest and events

Most museums, galleries, exhibitions, theatres, concert venues and places of interest in the UK offer discounted entry for VIPs.

Many sites also offer services to make their venue accessible to people with sight loss. A museum may offer guided tours or audio guides that your VIP can listen to as she moves amongst the exhibits. A concert venue may have special seats reserved that are closer to the stage. A theatre may provide audio-described performances. If your VIP is lucky, there may even be a chance to meet the cast and feel their costumes beforehand.

Contact the venue you're interested in visiting. Ask what discounts it can offer and what services it has to make your VIP's visit more enjoyable.

In conclusion

'It's not the winning but the taking part that is important'

There is so much truth in this statement. Being part of something that is bigger than oneself can help to make us who we are. It is the belonging, the social contacts, the pleasure of being with others, that makes us truly human.

I started this book by telling you of my failure many years ago when confronted by an old lady looking for hope on her 90th birthday.

You can help your VIP get back from a major trauma. If, with your help, she is now taking part in a social activity she enjoys, you will have given her back a proper life. You will know you've succeeded when she is relaxed in a social setting, and even laughing.

If you've managed that, congratulations. But don't let the skills you have picked up go to waste. Go out and find somebody else to coach. Lots of people would love to meet you. Well done on all you've achieved. We can both feel better about ourselves.

As a thank you for purchasing this book, I would like to offer you the opportunity to download an audio edition that your VIP can listen to and learn from directly.

To get your copy, please visit http://livingwithamd.co.uk/swatt123

xxxxxxxxxxxxxxxxxxxxxxxxxxxxxxxxxx

If you enjoyed reading this book and found it helpful, could I ask you to leave an honest review where you purchased it. It will encourage others to read it and get the same help.

xxxxxxxxxxxxxxxxxxxxxxxxxxxxxxxxxx

For the latest information on Macular degeneration please go to my web page www.livingwithamd.co.uk

Thank you
Paul Wallis

Lightning Source UK Ltd.
Milton Keynes UK
UKHW021901150222
398741UK00007B/315